Adding Insult to Injury

A review of the care of patients who died in hospital with a primary diagnosis of acute kidney injury (acute renal failure).

A report by the National Confidential Enquiry into Patient Outcome and Death (2009).

Compiled by:

J Stewart MB ChB LLM FRCP
Clinical Co-ordinator

G Findlay MB ChB FRCA
Clinical Co-ordinator

N Smith PhD
Clinical Researcher

K Kelly BA (Hons)
Research Assistant

M Mason PhD
Chief Executive

Contents

Acknowledgements

This report, published by NCEPOD, could not have been achieved without the support of a wide range of individuals and organisations.

Our particular thanks go to:

The expert group who advised NCEPOD:

Mr David Mitchell
Consultant Vascular Surgeon

Dr Andrew Lewington
Consultant Nephrologist

Dr Alastair Hutchison
Consultant Nephrologist

Dr Philip Kalra
Consultant Nephrologist

Dr Suren Kanagasundaram
Consultant Nephrologist

Professor Paul Roderick
Professor of Public Health Medicine

The advisors who reviewed the cases:

Dr Nihal Abosaif
Consultant Nephrologist and Acute Physician

Dr Reem Al-Jayyousi
Consultant Nephrologist

Dr Sunil Bhandari
Consultant Nephrologist and General Physician

Dr Sara Blakeley
Consultant Intensivist

Dr Emma Borthwick
Specialist Registrar in Nephrology and
Intensive Care Medicine

Dr Rachael Challiner
Consultant Intensivist and Nephrologist

Dr Andrew Davenport
Consultant Nephrologist

Dr Mark Devonald
Consultant Nephrologist

Dr John Dibble
Consultant Nephrologist

Dr Steve Dickinson
Specialist Registrar in Nephrology and
General Physician

Dr Alistair Douglas
Consultant in Acute Medicine and Nephrology

Dr Lui Forni
Consultant Nephrologist and Intensivist

Dr Andrew Gratrix
Consultant Intensivist and Anaesthetist

Dr Paul Johnston
Consultant Nephrologist

Dr Mike Jones
Consultant in Acute Medicine

Dr Nitin Kolhe
Consultant Nephrologist

Dr Paul Laboi
Consultant Nephrologist and General Physician

Dr Christopher Laing
Consultant Nephrologist

Dr Patrick MacDowall
Consultant Nephrologist and General Physician

Dr Stephen Morgan
Consultant Nephrologist

Dr Gareth Scholey
Specialist Registrar in Nephrology and
Intensive Care Medicine

Dr Christopher Thompson
Consultant Nephrologist and Intensivist

Dr Graham Warwick
Consultant Nephrologist

Dr Matthew Wise
Consultant Intensivist

The organisations that provided funding to cover the cost of this study:

National Patient Safety Agency
Department of Health, Social Services and
Public Safety (NI)
Aspen Healthcare
BMI Healthcare
Classic Hospitals
Covenant Healthcare Ltd
East Kent Medical Services Ltd
Fairfield Independent Hospital
HCA International
Hospital of St John and St Elizabeth
Isle of Man Health and Social Security Department
King Edward VII's Hospital Sister Agnes
Netcare Healthcare UK Ltd
New Victoria Hospital
Nuffield Health
Ramsay Health Care UK
Spire Health Care
St Anthony's Hospital
St Joseph's Hospital
States of Guernsey Board of Health
States of Jersey, Health and Social Services
The Benenden Hospital Trust
The Horder Centre
The Hospital Management Trust
The London Clinic
The London Oncology Clinic
Ulster Independent Clinic

The professional organisations that support our work and who constitute our Steering Group:

Association of Anaesthetists of Great Britain and Ireland
Association of Surgeons of Great Britain and Ireland
College of Emergency Medicine
Coroners' Society of England and Wales
Faculty of Dental Surgery of the Royal College of Surgeons of England
Faculty of Public Health of the Royal College of Physicians of the United Kingdom
Institute of Healthcare Management
Royal College of Anaesthetists
Royal College of Child Health and Paediatrics
Royal College of General Practitioners
Royal College of Nursing
Royal College of Obstetricians and Gynaecologists
Royal College of Ophthalmologists
Royal College of Pathologists
Royal College of Physicians of London
Royal College of Radiologists
Royal College of Surgeons of England

The authors and Trustees of NCEPOD would particularly like to thank the NCEPOD staff for their work in collecting and analysing the data for this study:

Robert Alleway, Sabah Begg, Maurice Blackman, Heather Cooper, Dolores Jarman, Rakhee Lakhani, Waqaar Majid, Eva Nwosu, Karen Protopapa and Hannah Shotton.

DISCLAIMER

This work was undertaken by NCEPOD, which received funding for this report from the National Patient Safety Agency. The views expressed in this publication are those of the authors and not necessarily those of the Agency.

Foreword

Recently a medical student was showing me her work. As a routine training exercise she had undertaken a case study of a hospital patient. From the hospital IT system, she had downloaded and tabulated the blood results and had devised a colour code for those falling outside the normal range. What caught my eye was a run of three to four days of blood results, urea and creatinine, printed in red. "Oh, that's the weekend" she sagely remarked.

What our report has revealed is that such patterns of deteriorating kidney function are all too common. Many of the examples could and should have been prevented. These episodes are being missed when they occur, and when discovered they are not always well treated. It is very standard medical care and the underlying principles are well known but merit spelling out in fairly basic terms.

In health, and quite unnoticed by us, the body is constantly keeping the essential control mechanism on an even keel. Entirely unconscious mechanisms make breath by breath adjustments so that oxygen, carbon dioxide and pH are all kept within narrow bounds. The heart pumps this quality controlled blood at a predetermined pressure. As we go through our daily cycles of exercise, digestion and rest the blood flow is adjusted according to the minute to minute needs of the body's various organs and tissues by a finely tuned network of blood vessels. The kidneys constantly filter the blood removing waste and making adjustments to sodium and potassium. These electrolytes are critical to the electrical charge across cell membranes: the biological battery that is gives power to the heart, muscles, brain and nerve cells and enables the functioning of every cell in the body. All of this is normal physiology: a complex, integrated autopilot that keeps us alive.

Failure of the heart or the lungs to maintain their life - sustaining roles is immediately evident but when the kidneys fail in their function it may go unnoticed. In part this happens because the body's mechanisms deceive us. When things start to go wrong in the course of illness, the body economises on blood flow. The hands and feet may be noticeably cold but more important and unseen, the blood flow to the kidneys is reduced. It takes hours before the changes are evident in the blood and days before it is clinically evident on external examination. By then there may be structural damage to the kidney at a cellular level, dubbed by kidney specialists as acute kidney injury - the term used in this report. Caught early transient malfunction can be reversed by prompt action but once established these changes are difficult to reverse and the integrated physiological mechanisms may be in a dangerous downward spiral.

Many of the dramatic presentations of acute illness - sepsis, haemorrhage, heart attack - can result in reduced blood flow to the kidneys but so can dehydration caused by vomiting, diarrhoea, intestinal obstruction or even simply not having the energy and mobility to drink. Being in hospital interrupts the usual daily routine of making cups of tea, which the patient might do if at home, and deliberate fasting before anaesthesia are examples of the many ways in which illness and the care of the ill can inadvertently add to the problem.

All of this is very well known. Underpinning all
clinical care is to do all the small things well: attend
to the pressure areas, prevent blood clots, maintain
nourishment and maintain hydration. It's absolutely basic
medicine. So what's happening? As we have got better
at treating serious illness and can offer really effective
treatments and operations, are we losing sight of the
basics? Is greater specialisation and loss of generalists
partly to blame? Is continuity of care suffering as we quite
properly give some outside life back to junior doctors?
Whatever it is we have to relearn the old lesson about
preventing, detecting, and managing acute kidney injury.
If a medical student can make the observation "Oh, that's
the weekend" it's time for us all to pay attention.

Professor T Treasure
NCEPOD Chairman

Principal recommendations

All patients admitted as an emergency, regardless of specialty, should have their electrolytes checked routinely on admission and appropriately thereafter. This will prevent the insidious and unrecognised onset of AKI. (Clinical Directors and Medical Directors)

Predictable and avoidable AKI should never occur. For those in-patients who develop AKI there should be both a robust assessment of contributory risk factors and an awareness of the possible complications that may arise. (Clinical Directors and Medical Directors)

All acute admissions should receive adequate senior reviews (with a consultant review within 12 hours of admission as previously recommended by NCEPOD[3]). (Clinical Directors and Medical Directors)

NCEPOD recommends that the guidance for recognising the acutely ill patient (NICE CG 50) is disseminated and implemented. In particular all acute patients should have admission physiological observations performed and a written physiological monitoring plan made, taking into account the degree of illness and risk of deterioration. (Clinical Directors and Medical Directors)

There should be sufficient critical care and renal beds to allow rapid step up in care if appropriate. (Department of Health)

All level 3 units should have the ability to deliver renal replacement therapy; and where appropriate these patients should receive clinical input from a nephrologist. (Clinical Directors and Medical Directors)

All acute admitting hospitals should have access to either onsite nephrologists or a dedicated nephrology service within reasonable distance of the admitting hospital. (Clinical Directors and Medical Directors)

All acute admitting hospitals should have access to a renal ultrasound scanning service 24 hours a day including the weekends and the ability to provide emergency relief of renal obstruction. (Clinical Directors and Medical Directors)

Introduction

Acute kidney injury (AKI), formerly known as acute renal failure, is both a prevalent and serious problem amongst hospitalised patients. Although no definitive studies have been undertaken in the UK the prevalence amongst hospitalised patients in the US is 4.9%[1]. Associated mortality rates have been wide ranging[2]. Clinically, AKI should be easily recognised by the onset of oliguria, anuria and/or deteriorating biochemistry. However, if unrecognised and allowed to deteriorate, AKI will result in uraemia, acidosis, hyperkalaemia and ultimately death.

Strategies to reduce the risk of AKI are well known; they include identifying relevant risk factors, appropriate monitoring of blood biochemistry, rapid remedial action when AKI occurs, and appropriate referral of patients to specialist services. However, it is unknown if these strategies are being implemented and many factors around patients with AKI, both amongst those admitted to and already within UK hospitals remain unclear.

Despite the seriousness of this condition, and its potential for treatment if detected early, it lacks a standard definition, and historically its treatment has been a matter of debate amongst clinicians. Recently, attempts have been made to classify AKI, as a set of functional criteria which give perspective on the degree of injury. To this end the RIFLE classification (risk, injury, failure, loss of kidney function, end-stage kidney disease) was devised and then further refined by the Acute Kidney Injury Network.

All hospital patients, regardless of specialty, are at risk of AKI either through their presenting illness or subsequent iatrogenic injury. However, it is unknown whether potential deficiencies in the care of patients with AKI are predominantly due to clinical failure (risk assessment, recognition, and management); or whether organisational issues such as a lack of availability of expert advice and intensive support are equally culpable. In addition, there exist treatments for AKI which are the result of historical dogma rather than evidence based therapeutics (e.g. diuretics/dopamine) and it is unclear to what extent these are still practised.

The aim of this study was to look in detail at these issues allowing NCEPOD to provide recommendations for the future care of patients with AKI.

1 - Method

Study aim

The primary aim of this study was to examine the process of care of patients who died in hospital with acute kidney injury (AKI), in order to identify remediable factors in the care received by these patients.

Expert group

A multidisciplinary group of experts comprising nephrologists, general surgeons, general physicians, anaesthetists, intensivists, an expert in clinical epidemiology/public health medicine and lay representatives contributed to the design of the study and reviewed the findings.

Objectives

The expert group identified seven main thematic areas that would address the overall aim of the study and these will be addressed throughout the following chapters:
- Diagnosis and recognition of AKI
- Recognition of risk factors associated with AKI
- Prevention of AKI
- Assessment of patients recognised as being in AKI
- Management of established AKI
- Recognition and management of complications of AKI
- Organisational factors relevant to the treatment of AKI

Hospital participation

National Health Service hospitals in England, Wales and Northern Ireland were expected to participate, as well as hospitals in the independent sector and public hospitals in the Isle of Man, Guernsey and Jersey.

Within each hospital, a named contact, referred to as the NCEPOD Local Reporter, acted as a liaison between NCEPOD and the hospital staff, facilitating case identification, dissemination of questionnaires and data collation.

Pilot study

A short exercise was conducted with the expert group to test the feasibility of using ICD10 coding for patient identification. Anonymised casenotes from a previous NCEPOD study on emergency admissions[3] were used to assess this. The casenotes of 20 patients coded for AKI (N17) were assessed by experts to confirm the clinical indication of AKI. Additionally, a selection of cases coded for sepsis (A41) and 50 randomly selected (non N17 or A41) cases were assessed to determine the incidence of AKI in these patients.

It was found that all of the cases coded for N17 were indicative of AKI. In addition a number of patients coded for sepsis had documented signs of AKI (7/20) or it was not possible to exclude AKI (10/20). The incidence of AKI in the randomly selected group was very low (2/50).

To help avoid unnecessary work by clinicians, the decision was made to only include cases coded with N17 in the main study sample.

Main study

Study population
Patients aged 16 years or older were eligible for inclusion if they were coded for a diagnosis of AKI and subsequently died in hospital between January 1st 2007 and March 31st 2007 inclusive.

Exclusion criteria

The following patient groups were excluded:
- Patients already on renal replacement therapy (RRT)
- Patients whose admission was, at the outset, for palliative care.

Case ascertainment

The NCEPOD Local Reporter identified all patients who died within their hospital(s) during the study period, regardless of disease type or disorder. The information requested for each case included the primary and secondary diagnosis codes and details of the clinician responsible for the patient at the time of death.

Questionnaires and casenotes

There were two questionnaires used to collect data for this study, one clinical questionnaire per patient and one organisational questionnaire per hospital.

1. Clinical Questionnaire

This questionnaire was sent to the consultant caring for the patient at the time of death. Information was requested concerning the recognition, assessment and management of AKI.

2. Organisational questionnaire

This questionnaire concerned data on the staff, facilities and protocols, relevant to the management of AKI, for each participating hospital. Information was collected at the hospital level as it provided a better indication of the facilities available for a patient at the location where they were receiving care, rather than all the facilities available within the Trust as a whole.

The organisational questionnaire was sent to the NCEPOD Local Reporter for completion in collaboration with relevant specialty input. Clinical questionnaires were either sent to the NCEPOD Local Reporter for dissemination or directly to the clinician involved.

However, whichever method was used, it was requested that the completed questionnaires were returned directly to NCEPOD to maintain confidentiality.

3. Casenotes

For each case to be peer reviewed photocopies of the following casenote extracts were requested:
- Inpatient annotations.
- Nursing notes.
- Biochemistry results (LFT, U&E).
- Drug charts.
- Fluid balance charts (including urine output).
- Observation charts (including TPR, CVP).
- Weight chart.
- Urinalysis.
- X-ray/CT/ultrasound results.
- Any operating notes.
- Do Not Attempt Resuscitation (DNAR) statement.
- Autopsy report.

Advisor group

A multidisciplinary group of advisors was recruited to review the casenotes and associated questionnaires. The group of advisors comprised clinicians from the following specialties: general medicine, nephrology and intensive care medicine.

All questionnaires and casenotes were anonymised by the non-clinical staff at NCEPOD. All patient, clinician and hospital identifiers were removed. Neither clinical co-ordinators at NCEPOD, nor the advisors had access to any identifiable information.

After being anonymised each case was reviewed by one advisor within a multidisciplinary group. At regular intervals throughout the meeting, the chair allowed a period of discussion for each advisor to summarise their cases and ask for opinions from other specialties or raise aspects of a case for discussion.

The following grading system was used by the advisors to grade the overall care each patient received.

Good practice: A standard that you would accept from yourself, your trainees and your institution.
Room for improvement: Aspects of clinical care that could have been better.
Room for improvement: Aspects of organisational care that could have been better.
Room for improvement: Aspects of both clinical and organisational care that could have been better.
Less than satisfactory: Several aspects of clinical and/or organisational care that were well below that you would accept from yourself, your trainees and your institution.
Insufficient information submitted to NCEPOD to assess the quality of care.

Quality and confidentiality

Each case was given a unique NCEPOD number so that cases could not easily be linked to a hospital.

The data from all questionnaires received were electronically scanned into a preset database. Prior to any analysis taking place, the data were cleaned to ensure that there were no duplicate records and that erroneous data had not been entered during scanning. Any fields that contained data that could not be validated were removed.

Data analysis

Following cleaning of the quantitative data, descriptive data summaries were produced.

The qualitative data collected from the advisors' opinions and free text answers in the clinical questionnaires were coded, where applicable, according to content to allow quantitative analysis. The data were reviewed by NCEPOD clinical co-ordinators to identify the nature and frequency of recurring themes.

Case studies have been used throughout this report to illustrate particular themes.

All data were analysed using Microsoft Access and Excel by the non-clinical staff at NCEPOD.

The findings of the report were reviewed by the expert group, advisors and the NCEPOD steering group prior to publication.

2 - Data returns

Clinical questionnaire returns

1518 patients from 215 hospitals were identified as
meeting the inclusion criteria for the study. Four hundred
and seventy three cases were subsequently excluded
from the study for either not being indicative of AKI, or
because the admission, at the outset, was for palliative
care. For a further 69 cases the casenotes were reported
as being lost or the consultant in charge of the patient
at the time of their death had left the Trust. For the
remaining 976 included patients, a clinical questionnaire
and/or casenotes was received for 700 cases (72%).

Study sample denominator data

Figure 2.1 shows that 645 (587 + 58) completed clinician
questionnaires were returned.

Figure 2.1 Data returns

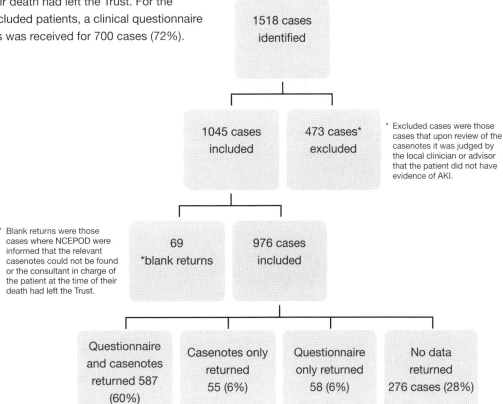

* Excluded cases were those
cases that upon review of the
casenotes it was judged by
the local clinician or advisor
that the patient did not have
evidence of AKI.

* Blank returns were those
cases where NCEPOD were
informed that the relevant
casenotes could not be found
or the consultant in charge of
the patient at the time of their
death had left the Trust.

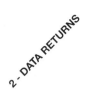

Upon review of the casenotes it was found that 61 patients had undergone an inter hospital transfer and for a further 17 cases the casenote extracts were very incomplete. It should be noted that for the transferred patients, only notes from the receiving hospital were submitted to NCEPOD, hence these cases could not be assessed by the advisors. Therefore 564 cases (642 – 61 – 17) were included in the peer review process.

A completed clinician questionnaire was received for 645 patients. Fifty three of the 645 completed questionnaires were for patients who were documented as being an inter-hospital transfer (Table 2.1). These cases have been excluded from subsequent analysis as no information from the transferring hospital was available.

For this reason the denominator will change depending on whether data were used from the clinical questionnaire, the advisor opinion or a combination of the two.

Table 2.1 Type of admission (clinical questionnaire)

Type of admission	Number of patients (%)
An emergency	570 (90)
Inter-hospital transfer	53 (9)
A planned admission	8 (1)
Subtotal	631
Not answered	14
Total	645

A completed organisational questionnaire was received from 305 hospitals and this was therefore the denominator for the analysis of organisational factors, in relation to AKI management.

Sample limitations

When reading this report it will become apparent that the method of patient identification (i.e. ICD10 coding) did not capture many post-surgical patients. This finding was discussed with the expert group and advisors, whom, from their own experiences of managing AKI, expected more surgical patients. The conclusion reached by the experts/advisors was that these patients are probably coded for a condition related to the surgical procedure they received, rather than AKI. NCEPOD realises the importance of looking at the care of this group of patients and will address this in a future study which is due for publication in late 2010 (concentrating on emergency and elective surgery in the elderly).

A second important subset of patients that have not been assessed in this study are those patients who had an inter-hospital transfer (see above).

3 - Study population and overall quality of care

Study population

There was an even split between males and females (48% vs 52%) in this study. The median age was 83 with a range of 39 – 102 years (see Figure 3.1).

The predilection towards the elderly was unsurprising in view of their vulnerability to renal injury from age-related reduction in glomerular filtration rate (GFR), medication and intercurrent illness.

The majority (570/631) of patients were admitted as emergencies (Table 2.1) which given the nature of AKI is understandable; its onset being insidious and often silent until overt ill health or complications become manifest.

Number of patients

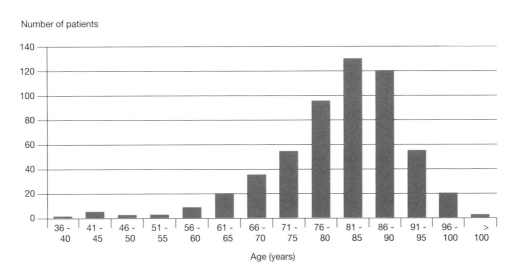

Figure 3.1 Age distribution of study population

Number of patients

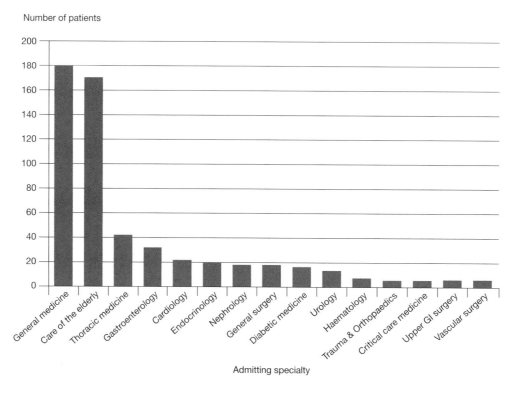

Admitting specialty

Figure 3.2 Specialties of admitting consultants

There was a broad spectrum of admitting specialties and these are outlined in Figure 3.2. The majority of cases were admitted to medical specialties which given the commonest presentations of AKI (deterioration in health, abnormal biochemistry) was not unexpected. As previously mentioned in Chapter 2, a paucity of patients was admitted to surgery. Additionally this may reflect that the majority of surgical patients die either when an operation has been precluded owing to poor prognosis, or following post-operative complications. However, in both these scenarios the primary cause of death is not acute kidney injury but either an inoperable or post-operative problem with AKI secondary to it; such cases would not have been identified during sampling. Furthermore, the advisors found that only 10/107 patients were cases of post-operative AKI. This might suggest that most post-operative AKI was either treated successfully or was not recorded as the primary cause of death.

The distribution of day of admission is illustrated in Figure 3.3. As can be seen the frequency of admissions was higher during the working week compared to weekend admissions.

Table 3.1 Kidney disease status on admission

Evidence of kidney disease on admission	Number of patients (%)
Yes	515 (88)
No	69 (12)
Subtotal	584
Not answered	8
Total	592

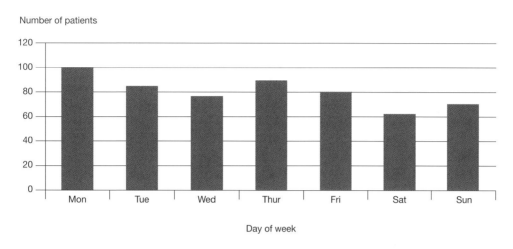

Number of patients

Day of week

Figure 3.3 Day on which the study patients were admitted

Table 3.2 Type of kidney disease diagnosed on admission

Type of kidney disease	Number of patients (%)
A new diagnosis	216 (46)
Chronic	74 (16)
Acute on Chronic	182 (38)
Subtotal	**472**
Not answered	43
Total	**515**

Table 3.3 Definitive diagnosis for AKI

Definitive diagnosis for AKI	Number of patients (%)
Yes	293 (65)
No	155 (35)
Subtotal	**448**
Not answered	144
Total	**592**

Information from the clinician questionnaire revealed that 515/584 (88%) patients had evidence of kidney disease on admission (Table 3.1). In 216/472 (46%) patients this was a new diagnosis; 74/472 (16%) had chronic kidney disease and 182/472 (38%) acute on chronic kidney disease. The type of kidney disease was not indicated for 43 patients (Table 3.2). For those without kidney disease on admission only 10/69 (14%) had the pursuant risk of renal disease documented.

Data from the clincial questionnaire indicated that 65% (293/448) of patients had a definitive diagnosis made to explain their AKI, this question was not answered for 144 cases (Table 3.3). By far the commonest definitive diagnoses for AKI was dehydration/hypovolaemia/volume depletion either as a sole diagnosis or coupled with a secondary diagnosis (e.g sepsis).

In addition clinicians stated that for 73/539 (14%) of patients the AKI was avoidable (Table 3.4). It should be noted that this included a number of patients who presented to hospital dehydrated with AKI, where the clinician was of the opinion that perhaps greater fluid intake in the community would have prevented the subsequent deterioration and development of AKI.

Table 3.4 Clinicians' opinion on whether the patients' AKI was avoidable

AKI avoidable	Number of patients (%)
Yes	73 (14)
No	466 (86)
Subtotal	539
Not answered	53
Total	592

Overall quality of care

The advisors were asked to comment on the overall quality of clinical care received by the patients in the study (Figure 3.4). As can be seen only 50% of patients were considered to have received an overall standard of care that was considered good. The majority of patients who received less than good care were more often judged to have room for improvement in clinical rather than organisational care; suggesting deficiencies in AKI care are primarily related to the clinicians managing those patients and not deficiencies in process or material. This may indicate a lack of awareness of the inherent risk of AKI amongst hospitalised patients; a poor understanding of the pathophysiology of the condition; or inadequate knowledge of its management amongst medical staff. It is likely this reflects deficiencies in training, both at undergraduate and postgraduate level, which is of particular note considering the prevalence and clinical importance of AKI.

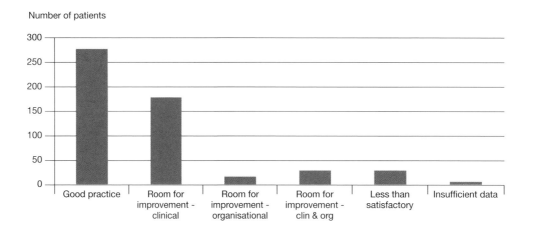

Figure 3.4 Overall assessment of care – advisors' opinion

When the overall quality of care within the study group was further broken down into those who developed AKI pre- and post-admission it can be seen that there was far more evidence of less than good practice in the post-admission AKI patients (Figure 3.5); with only a third (34/107) receiving good care as judged by the advisors.

Again, the majority of the deficiencies were in clinical care. There needs to be raised awareness amongst doctors about the risk of developing AKI as an inpatient and more education of doctors around the precipitants and management of patients who do subsequently develop AKI.

Number of patients

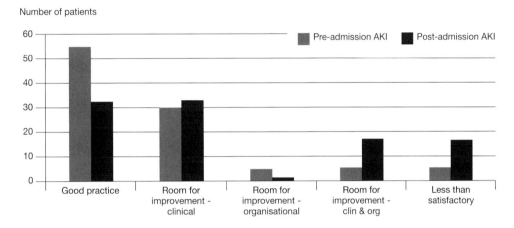

Figure 3.5 Overall assessment of care (pre-admission vs post-admission AKI)

n = 457 and 107 for pre- and post-admission AKI respectively

4 - Admission and assessment of acute kidney injury

Good clinical assessment is the bedrock of competent and focused clinical practice and should be a uniform skill amongst clinicians. This holds true regardless of grade, and to this end adequate supervision is required. Moreover, it is not sufficient for a doctor to simply appreciate the possible diagnoses; they should also be able to recognise and record when a patient is acutely unwell. As such Modified Early Warning Scores (MEWS) (Appendix 5) have been devised and instituted in many acute hospitals.

With these issues in mind, the grade of the doctor who first admitted the patient was reviewed.

As shown in Table 4.1 the majority of patients were clerked by junior staff; the commonest admitting grade being SHO/ST1-2 or below. When the grade of admitting doctor was compared with the overall quality of care of the patient it can be seen that the more senior the admitting doctor the more likely it was that their total hospital episode will have been judged to have been of a better standard of care (Table 4.2).

Table 4.1 Grade of doctor undertaking initial clerking

Grade of doctor	Number of patients
FY1	101
FY2	83
SHO/ST1-2	257
SpR/ST3 or higher	79
Staff Grade	13
Consultant	11
Other	16
Subtotal	**560**
Not answered	32
Total	**592**

Table 4.2 Grade of doctor undertaking initial clerking versus overall quality of care

Overall assessment of care - advisors' opinion	FY1, FY2 or SHO/ST1-2	SpR/ST3 or higher
Good practice	173 (47)	46 (65)
Room for improvement - clinical	122 (33)	16 (23)
Room for improvement - organisational	10 (3)	3 (4)
Room for improvement - clinical & organisational	32 (9)	4 (6)
Less than satisfactory	29 (8)	2 (3)
Total	**366**	**71**

The above data are from those cases for which an advisor assessment form and clinical questionnaire was completed.

It would be preferable that juniors were all supervised such that the same standard of care was achieved regardless of the admitting doctor. This has previously been highlighted in a report on emergency admissions, which commented on the possibility of a causal association between the quality of the initial assessment and the overall quality of care of a patient's admission[3].

The advisors were asked whether the patient's illness severity was recognised (Table 4.3).

Table 4.3 Recognition of the severity of the patients' illness

Severity of patients' illness recognised	Number of patients (%)
Yes	421 (84)
No	81 (16)
Subtotal	502
Insufficient data	62
Total	564

In their opinion, 81/502 (16%) did not have the severity of their illness recognised. The specific use of MEWS (or similar) in the assessment of the patients was reviewed.

Table 4.4 Evidence of MEWS in place

MEWS in place	Number of patients (%)
Yes	228 (55)
Yes but score not documented	42 (10)
No	146 (35)
Subtotal	416
Insufficient data	148
Total	564

It was found that 146/416 (35%) patients did not have MEWS available for patient assessment; however 42/416 (10%) did have MEWS but these were not used (Table 4.4). Moreover, 10/42 patients not only did not have their illness severity recognised but also did not have MEWS recorded even though they were available. There appeared to be slightly better recognition of severity of illness when SpR/ST3s performed the initial assessment (Table 4.5)

Table 4.5 Illness severity recognition versus grade of assessor

Grade of initial assessor	Severity of illness recognised	
	Yes (%)	No (%)
FY1	61 (79)	16 (21)
FY2	53 (82)	12 (18)
SHO/ST1-2	153 (84)	30 (16)
SPR/ST3 or higher	61 (94)	4 (6)
Staff grade	7 (78)	2 (22)
Consultant	6 (86)	1 (14)
Total	341	65

The above data are from those cases for which an advisor assessment form and clinician questionnaire was completed.

The following case study illustrates a lack of appreciation of both illness severity and poor diagnostic skills.

Case study 1

An elderly patient was admitted to an Emergency Department with a history of dyspnoea and AKI. Their past medical history included congestive cardiac failure and diabetes for which the patient was taking metformin. Initial investigations showed a white cell count of 25; arterial blood gas analysis revealing a pH of 6.98 and base excess of -25.The patient was treated as a case of left ventricular failure with diuretics and CPAP; subsequently dying within 12 hours of admission. There was no consideration as to whether the patient was septic or had lactic acidosis related to metformin.

The advisors believed that this was an example of poor management and a complete failure to recognise the possibility of sepsis and/or lactic acidosis both on clinical signs and biochemical results.

The effective management of AKI requires timely recognition that the problem exists; allowing risk factors to be reduced and remedial management implemented. Table 4.6 shows the advisors opinion as to whether there had been an unacceptable delay in the recognition of AKI for all patients and for those where the AKI developed pre-admission or post-admission. When the study cohort was analysed as a whole it was found that there was delayed recognition in 12% (64/542) of patients. Further analysis revealed that there was a marked difference in the frequency of delayed recognition depending on whether the patient was admitted with AKI or developed it post-admission; 5% (22/444) versus 43% (42/98) respectively. Whilst the total number of post-admission AKI patients was small it is reasonable to assert that patients should not be left a hostage to fortune; AKI is easily identified if clinicians are alive to its prevalence and undertake simple clinical observations and biochemistry to identify its presence. All patients admitted as an emergency should have their electrolytes checked on admission but more importantly appropriately thereafter; especially in those who are acutely unwell or at risk of AKI.

Table 4.6 Advisors opinion on delays in recognition, pre- vs post-admission AKI

Unacceptable delay	Pre-admission (%)	Post-admission (%)	Total (%)
Yes	22 (5)	42 (43)	64 (12)
No	422 (95)	56 (57)	478 (88)
Subtotal	444	98	542
Insufficient data	13	9	22
Total	457	107	564

Risk assessment

AKI is a condition that occurs when a patient with or without pre-existing renal disease is challenged by one or more well recognised renal insults. Thus of particular importance in the assessment of the patient who presents with AKI is consideration of factors that put them at risk of the condition. Ten risk factors had been identified by the Expert Group as being of the most importance when assessing a patient's risk of having or developing AKI (Table 4.7).

NCEPOD asked the clinicians completing the questionnaire whether these risk factors had been assessed and recorded in the patient's casenotes on admission. Only 16/588 (3%) patients had had all ten risk factors assessed and documented (Figure 4.1).

Table 4.7 Expert group 'top ten' risk factors

	AKI risk factor
1	Age
2	Co-morbidity
3	Medication
4	Previous chronic kidney disease
5	Hypovolaemia
6	Sepsis
7	Biochemistry
8	Urinalysis
9	Weight
10	Nutritional status

Number of patients

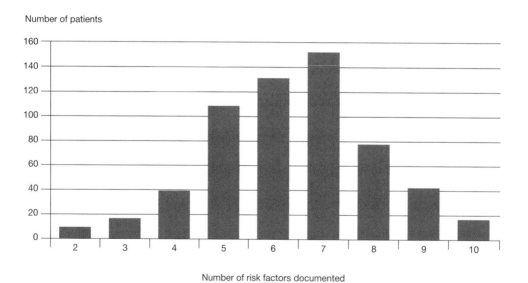

Number of risk factors documented

Figure 4.1 Frequency of documentation of key risk factors

In the opinion of the advisors 152/518 (29%) patients did not have an adequate assessment or documentation of the most important risk factors for AKI; with inadequate assessment of risk factors in 24% (99/419) of those patients admitted with AKI and 54% (53/99) of those who developed AKI post-admission (Table 4.8).

Table 4.8 Adequacy of AKI risk assessment, pre- vs post-admission AKI

Adequate risk assessment	Pre-admission (%)	Post-admission (%)	Total
Yes	320 (76)	46 (46)	366 (71)
No	99 (24)	53 (54)	152 (29)
Subtotal	419	99	518
Insufficient data	38	8	46
Total	457	107	564

The advisors found that the commonest risk factors not assessed were medication, co-morbidity and hypovolaemia (Table 4.9) That such basic risk factors should be overlooked in a large proportion of patients is a serious issue and further evidence of the poor understanding of the pathophysiology. The management of AKI is often primarily dependant on risk factors being identified and removed, and for euvolaemia to be restored. For these to be overlooked suggests that the basics of AKI management are either ignored by, or unknown to, many clinicians.

Table 4.9 Inadequate assessment of risk factors

Risk factor	Number of patients
Medication	66
Hypovolaemia	60
Sepsis	59
Co-morbidity	56
Urinalysis	54
Hypotension	52
Age	42
Previous chronic kidney disease	37
Nutritional status	36
Biochemistry	30
Weight	28

Answers may be multiple for the 152 patients that advisors believed had an inadequate assessment of risk factors for AKI

The following case study illustrates the importance of basic management.

Case study 2

An elderly patient was admitted with a fractured neck of femur. The patient was known to have chronic kidney disease but the electrolytes on admission showed no evidence of recent deterioration. The patient was noted to be taking aspirin and two diuretics. Hemi-arthroplasty was undertaken but post-operatively the patient developed worsening renal function consistent with pre-renal failure. Whilst this was noted and recorded, the diuretics were not discontinued and the patient was given inadequate intravenous fluid replacement. Renal function continued to deteriorate to the point where significant acidosis developed. After a prolonged hospital stay the patient ultimately died of AKI secondary to hypovolaemia precipitated by the above mismanagement.

The advisors felt that this case illustrated both poor understanding of pre-renal failure and a marked lack of clinical care.

Of the cases assessed by the advisors 54/152 (36%) patients, judged to have had an inadequate risk assessment for AKI, did not have urinalysis performed; of these, 46/99 were admitted with AKI and 8/53 developed AKI post-admission. Whilst urinalysis may be of limited use in some AKI scenarios it is notable that such a basic and obvious investigation of renal dysfunction should be omitted in such a high proportion of patients. There was however a discrepancy between the clinicians and the advisors with the clinicians claiming 150 patients did not have urinalysis. This suggests that the problem is more prevalent than the advisors were able to appreciate. The advisors remarked on the fact that such basic parameters of AKI risk were being overlooked. As a common problem within hospitals, risk assessment of AKI should be both intuitive and robust.

Case study 3

An elderly patient was admitted to hospital with cardiac failure and renal dysfunction. They were found to be in renal failure on admission. Over the following 35 days the renal function continued to deteriorate eventually necessitating transfer to a specialist unit. It was only on arrival at this unit that the patient's urine was tested by dipstick and found to contain significant protein and blood.

Advisors believed that management would have been improved by urine dipstick on admission.

Renal disease and diagnoses

Table 4.10 Type of kidney disease diagnosed on admission

Type of renal disease	Number of patients (%)
A new diagnosis	216 (46)
Chronic	74 (16)
Acute on Chronic	182 (39)
Subtotal	**472**
Not answered	43
Total	**515**

Of all the patients included in the study, 88% (515/584) had evidence of renal disease on admission (Table 3.1). Of these, 46% (216/472) were acute kidney injury with no history suggestive of pre-existing chronic kidney disease (Table 4.10). Of those who had pre-existing renal disease, 71% (182/256) were acute on chronic renal disease and 29% (74/256) had chronic kidney disease. The aetiology of the pre-existing chronic kidney disease was extremely broad although the most prevalent diagnoses were the usual suspects of hypertension and diabetes. For a large proportion, the aetiology was either unknown or not recorded.

Table 4.11 AKI stage on recognition

AKI stage	Pre-admission AKI Number of patients (%)	Post-admission AKI Number of patients (%)	Total Number of patients (%)
1	52 (14)	26 (26)	78 (16)
2	75 (20)	39 (39)	114 (24)
3	256 (67)	35 (35)	291 (60)
Total	**383**	**100**	**483**

Percentage of group

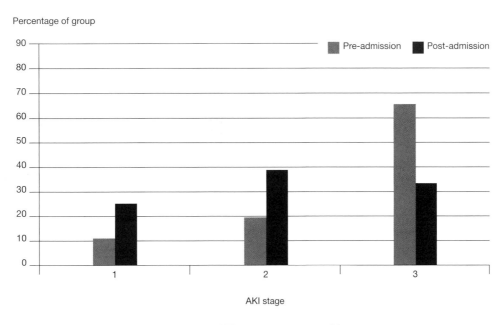

AKI stage

Figure 4.2 AKI stage on recognition

The advisors were asked what stage AKI the patients were in at the time their renal failure was diagnosed. Table 4.11 shows the proportion of patients in stages 1-3 (Appendix 3). In total 60% (291/483) of all the patients in the study were in stage 3 AKI when their renal failure was recognised. The data were further analysed to look at the stage of AKI of those who presented in renal failure against those who developed it post-admission: 74% (74/100) of patients who developed AKI post-admission were in stage 2/3 AKI at the time their renal injury was recognised (Figure 4.2 and Table 4.11). It is a matter of debate whether the stage of AKI in those admitted in renal failure is of any great import when studying the management of this condition. However, it was of concern that three quarters of patients who developed AKI as inpatients in this study were allowed to progress to the more severe end of the AKI spectrum before recognition and appropriate management was initiated. Especially in view of the clear links that have been made between increasing AKI stage and worsening mortality.

The clinicians were asked if a definitive diagnosis was made during the admission to explain the AKI. In the opinion of the clinicians, 64% (290/450) had a definitive diagnosis made. The advisors were also asked whether a definitive diagnosis was made to explain the AKI. In their opinion 300 patients had a definitive diagnosis made; however it was their opinion that in 43/300 (14%) the diagnosis was incorrect. The commonest incorrect diagnoses were hypotension and hypovolaemia. For these patients the advisors believed there was generally additional pathology to explain the aetiology of the AKI. It is perhaps fairer to suggest that this indicates incomplete rather than incorrect diagnoses. It is important for clinicians to recognise that AKI may be multi-factorial and shouldn't be attributed solely to the most obvious cause. As previously alluded to it is a matter of education and training that clinicians are reminded of the pathophysiology of this important condition.

Table 4.12 Predictability/avoidability of post-admission AKI

	Avoidable	Unavoidable	Not specified	Total
Predictable	22	22	21	65
Unpredictable	-	11	7	18
Not specified	11	4	9	24
Total	**33**	**37**	**37**	**107**

In those patients who developed AKI post-admission the advisors were asked whether the ensuing AKI was either predictable and/or avoidable. Table 4.12 shows the results of this analysis. Overall cases of AKI, 65/107 were considered predictable and 33/107 avoidable; 22/107 predictable but avoidable; 22/107 predictable but unavoidable; 11/107 unpredictable and unavoidable. These figures suggest that the prevalence of AKI may be higher than necessary as clinicians are not alive to the possibility that AKI may ensue. Furthermore, for 21% (22/107) of patients that developed AKI as an inpatient in this study, all of whom died of AKI, the renal insult was both foreseeable and avoidable. It seems then that patients died unnecessarily from renal disease when forethought and management would have avoided this. This suggests that consideration ought to be given to bedside screening protocols to detect those patients who are at risk of renal injury.

Complications of AKI

Established AKI can result in serious, life-threatening complications. The advisors found evidence in the casenotes that 465/564 (83%) of patients in this study suffered one or more complication of AKI. The commonest occurring complications were found to be acidosis, hyperkalaemia and sepsis (Figure 4.3). However, the advisors found that in 55/436 (13%) cases one or more complications were not recognised (Table 4.13); the commonest missed complications being acidosis and sepsis (Figure 4.4); in addition it was noted that patients with hyperkalaemia and respiratory failure were also being missed. Thus there is evidence that even the commonest complications were being overlooked.

Complications should be anticipated and avoided where possible. In the opinion of the advisors 74/431 complications were avoidable (Table 4.14).

Table 4.13 Recognition of the complications of AKI – Advisors' opinion

Complications of AKI recognised	Number of patients (%)
Yes	381 (87)
No	55 (13)
Subtotal	**436**
Insufficient data	29
Total	**465**

Table 4.14 Avoidable complications of AKI – Advisors' opinion

Complications of AKI avoidable	Number of patients (%)
Yes	74 (17)
No	357 (83)
Subtotal	**431**
Insufficient data	34
Total	**465**

Number of patients

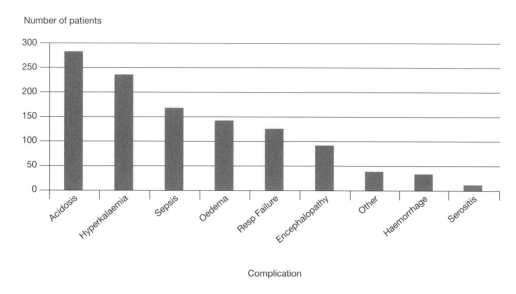

Complication

Figure 4.3 Complications of AKI

Number of patients

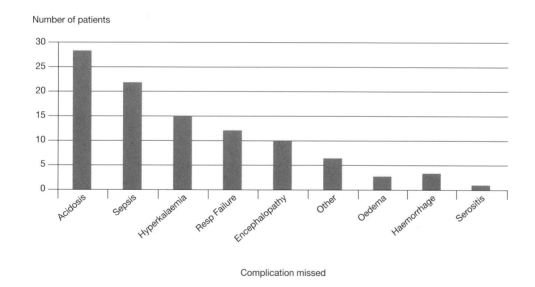

Complication missed

Figure 4.4 Missed complications – advisors' opinion in the 55 cases highlighted in Table 4.13

Table 4.15 Management of the complications of AKI – Advisors' opinion

Appropriate management of AKI	Number of patients (%)
Yes	334 (78)
No	94 (22)
Subtotal	**428**
Insufficient data	37
Total	**465**

Complications should not only be recognised but treated appropriately; however in the advisors' opinion 94/428 (22%) complications were managed inappropriately (Table 4.15). It is alarming that patients in this study died with evidence of unrecognised serious complications; and that some of these complications should have been foreseen and proactively avoided. If these complications had been recognised it is entirely possible that the outcome might have been different. The basic tenets of AKI management should not be the sole preserve of physicians and nephrologists, but a well rehearsed part of every hospital doctor's clinical armoury. As AKI can affect all hospital patients regardless of specialty a broad brush approach should be taken to postgraduate training in this area.

The management of AKI requires senior input in order to reduce morbidity, facilitate appropriate investigations and reduce complications. Leaving complex and potentially reversible management problems to junior staff alone is always unacceptable. This applies to AKI as much as any other condition. In the advisors opinion, 25% (see Chapter 8) of patients in this study had inadequate senior review. As can be seen above there was evidence of avoidable renal injury and/or complications occurring in a substantial proportion of patients and this percentage may have been reduced with better senior input.

Case study 4

An elderly patient was admitted with a short history of abdominal pain and distension. Initial assessment showed them to be hypotensive with marked abdominal distension, a white cell count of 29 and C-reactive protein of 80. There was evidence of renal dysfunction with a urea of 19 mmol/l and creatinine of 192 micromol/l. Following admission the patient was repeatedly reviewed by junior medical staff but despite a deteriorating clinical condition was not reviewed by a senior doctor and died within 24 hours of arrival.

Advisors were concerned about the lack of senior review in a patient with persistent hypotension and likely sepsis.

Furthermore, many patients with complicated or resistant AKI will require referral to nephrologists for advice on further management. There was documented evidence that 31% (173/561) of patients in this study were referred; however in the advisors opinion a further 19% (77/379) should have been referred who were not. Of those who were referred 22% (35/167) were considered to have been referred late (see Chapter 3).

Key Findings

Only 50% (280/564) of AKI care was considered good by the advisors.

There was poor assessment of risk factors for AKI; both in the assessment of patients in established AKI and those who subsequently developed it.

The advisors judged there to be an unacceptable delay in recognising post-admission AKI in 43% (42/98) of patients.

A fifth (22/107) of post-admission AKI was both predictable and avoidable in the view of the advisors.

In the advisors' opinion complications of AKI were missed in 13% of cases (55/436), avoidable in 17% (74/431) and managed badly in 22% (94/428) of cases.

Recommendations

Initial clerking of all emergency patients should include a risk assessment for AKI. (Clinical Directors and Medical Directors)

All patients admitted as an emergency, regardless of specialty, should have their electrolytes checked routinely on admission and appropriately thereafter. This will prevent the insidious and unrecognised onset of AKI. (Clinical Directors and Medical Directors)

Predictable and avoidable AKI should never occur. For those in-patients who develop AKI there should be both a robust assessment of contributory risk factors and an awareness of the possible complications that may arise. (Clinical Directors and Medical Directors)

Undergraduate medical training should include the recognition of the sick patient and the prevention, diagnosis and management of AKI. (Deaneries)

Postgraduate training for all specialties should include awareness, causes, recognition, management and complications of AKI. (Deaneries)

5 - Investigation and management of acute kidney injury

Acute kidney injury (AKI) is most frequently caused by an ischaemic, septic or toxic insult to the kidney and only a small fraction of cases are caused by other intrinsic renal diseases such as acute interstitial nephritis or acute glomerulonephritis. Patients who develop AKI after admission to hospital often have multiple risk factors and the cause is frequently multi-factorial.

Assessment of the patient with AKI therefore starts with a careful history and examination, including a thorough evaluation of the patient's notes and drug treatment records where available. A focused history should identify pre-existing risk factors and potential causes for AKI including reduced fluid intake and/or increased fluid losses, urinary tract symptoms and recent drug ingestion. Clinical examination must include assessment of volume status. Palpation for a distended bladder - usually resulting from urinary retention in elderly men secondary to enlarged prostate - is also essential.

A baseline set of laboratory investigations should be sent including urinalysis, biochemistry, haematology and microbiology (urine culture ± blood culture) with more specific renal investigations being dependent upon the clinical presentation. Further investigations may include ECG, chest x-ray, and renal tract ultrasound.

Proper patient assessment and investigation will allow identification of those at risk for AKI, quantification of degree of AKI and assessment of progression or resolution of renal disease. A diagnosis may often be made after clinical evaluation, assessment of volume status and simple urinalysis, supplemented by renal imaging.

Table 5.1 Adequacy of the investigation of AKI

Adequate investigation of AKI	Number of patients (%)
Yes	362 (67)
No	178 (33)
Subtotal	**540**
Insufficient data	24
Total	**564**

Table 5.1 shows that in the opinion of the advisors 33% (178/540) of patients did not have adequate investigation of AKI.

Table 5.2 Omitted investigation of AKI – Advisors' opinion

Omitted from investigations	Number of patients
Ultrasound	94
Acid base balance	83
Volume status	76
Urinalysis	73
Early warning score	57
Sepsis recognition	48
Biochemistry	33
Other	18
TPR	16
Immunology	10
CT	5
Radioisotopes	1
Renal biopsy	1
Total	**515**

Table 5.2 shows the omissions recorded in the 178 patients who had an inadequate investigation. There were 515 omissions noted, an average of almost three omissions per patient. What is particularly notable is that many of these omissions were very basic tests and clinical findings. Very few of the omissions could be ascribed to lack of resources or provision of diagnostic equipment and appear to be due to lack of application of basic good medical practice.

Seventy three patients did not have simple urinalysis. This information can help greatly in the search for the cause of AKI. Not performing urinalysis or performing it late after admission can miss vital pointers to the pathology causing renal disease. Figure 5.1 highlights the importance of urinalysis. This is an extract from 'Diagnostic Evalutions of the Patient with Acute Renal Failure'[4].

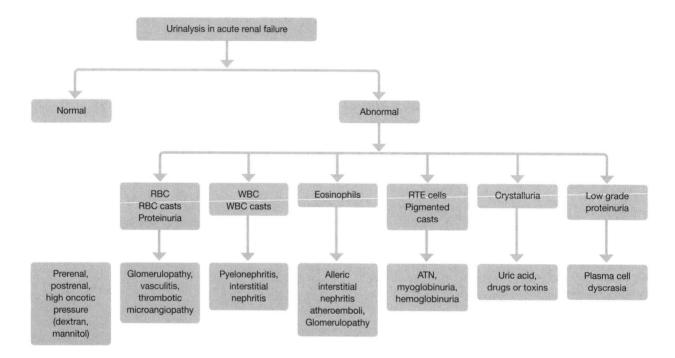

Figure 5.1. Urinalysis in AKI. *A normal urinalysis suggests a prerenal or postrenal form of AKI; however, many patients with AKI of postrenal causes have some cellular elements on urinalysis. Relatively uncommon causes of AKI that usually present with oligoanuria and a normal urinalysis are mannitol toxicity and large doses of dextran infusion. In these disorders, a "hyperoncotic state" occurs in which glomerular capillary oncotic pressure, combined with the intratubular hydrostatic pressure, exceeds the glomerular capillary hydrostatic pressure and stop glomerular filtration. Red blood cells (RBCs) can be seen with all renal forms of AKI. When RBC casts are present, glomerulonephritis or vasculitis is most likely. White blood cells (WBCs) can also be present in small numbers in the urine of patients with AKI.*

Large numbers of WBCs and WBC casts strongly suggest the presence of either pyelonephritis or acute interstitial nephritis. Eosinolphiluria (Hansel's stain) is often present in either allergic interstitial nephritis or atheroembolic disease. Renal tubular epithelial (RTE) cells and casts and pigmented granular casts typically are present in pigmenturia-associated AKI and in established acute tubular necrosis (ATN).

The presence of large numbers of crystals on urinalysis, in conjunction with the clinical history, may suggest uric acid, sulfonamides, or protease inhibitors as a cause of the renal failure.

All acute admissions to hospital should have reagent strip urinalysis and urine microscopy should be performed where reagent strip urinalysis is abnormal or patients are noted to have AKI. However a delay in performing urine microscopy may reduce the usefulness of the investigation as cellular elements are lost unless it is performed without undue delay. In addition the reduced skills in performing urine microscopy may contribute to this problem. However, if microscopy is to provide contributory information then it must be a fresh sample, microscoped promptly by someone with appropriate expertise.

Without simple tests such as biochemistry (33 cases) and acid base balance (83 cases) assessment it is impossible to quantify the degree of renal dysfunction and severity of physiological derangement.

AKI as a consequence of obstructive uropathy can be rapidly reversible if diagnosed and treated promptly. Ultrasound assessment of the renal tract is often considered first line investigation to rule this out. However in 94 cases there was no ultrasound performed, despite the advisors opinion that this was required. This may have been related to lack of clinical knowledge about importance of ultrasound in the initial evaluation of patients with AKI or may have been related to the availability of this investigation (see Chapter 9).

The lack of assessment of volume status, sepsis recognition and recording of simple measures (pulse, blood pressure and respiratory rate) is a major deficit in the assessment of any ill patient and is an obstacle to recognition of patients who are at high risk of deterioration. These simple assessments should be core to all health staff caring for inpatients.

Case study 5

An elderly patient presented to the medical take with a history of lethargy and confusion for a few days. It was noted on admission that the patient had AKI (urea 62mmol/l, creatinine 668micromol/l). A urinary catheter was inserted; however after initially draining 200mls there was no further urine output. There was no clear working diagnosis and a plan to modify existing drug therapy (to stop potential nephrotoxins) and volume resuscitate the patient was made. No further investigations were ordered. Twenty four hours later urea and creatinine had worsened despite the above treatment. Following consultant review a renal ultrasound was ordered. This revealed bilateral hydronephroses. Prior to decompression of the renal tract the patient suffered a cardiac arrest and died.

The advisors commented that the delay in imaging the renal tract may have contributed to death and that earlier intervention may have allowed recovery of renal function.

Deficiencies in the recognition of ill patients have been identified for many years and the care of the acutely ill hospitalised patient presents problems for health services worldwide[5]. Many studies have identified suboptimal care[6-8] which is frequently related to poor management of simple aspects of acute care – those involving the patient's airway, breathing and circulation, oxygen therapy, fluid balance and monitoring. Other contributory factors include organisation failures, a lack of knowledge, failure to appreciate the clinical urgency of a situation, a lack of supervision, failure to seek advice and poor communication. We have, yet again, found such basic deficiencies in patient care in this study and the challenge is how to reverse this deficit.

Case study 6

An elderly patient presented to hospital with a five day history of severe diarrhoea. Initial physiological observations were blood pressure 95/55mmHg, pulse 135 bpm, temperature 37.9° C. There was no record of respiratory rate or urine output. There was no record of an assessment of volaemic status. Over the next 48 hours observations were repeated eight times and revealed persistent hypotension, tachycardia and, on the four occasions where it was measured, tachypnoea. No urinary catheter was inserted. Biochemistry performed 48 hours after admission showed urea 33mmol/l, creatinine 455micromol/l and a severe metabolic acidosis. Despite eventual escalation of care to include critical care admission and renal replacement therapy the patient did not recover.

The advisors believed that there were long delays in recognition of signs of acute illness that prevented the provision of timely and appropriate care. The use of a track and trigger system (e.g. MEWS – Modified Early Warning Score) may have prevented these delays.

Management of AKI

AKI is potentially fatal but in many cases reversible when appropriately managed. Good practice suggests that people with AKI should be identified promptly and investigated to establish whether their kidney injury is caused by a condition requiring specific, specialist therapy (e.g. glomerulonephritis, vasculitis, haemolytic ureamic syndrome), or is the result of systemic disease such as infection, heart failure or hypovolaemia/ hypotension. Use of medicines known to damage the kidneys may need to be discontinued.

Published series of AKI suggest that up to 30% of cases may be preventable, with a further significant percentage potentially remediable through simple interventions such as volume repletion, discontinuing and/or avoiding certain potentially nephrotoxic agents, and earlier recognition of conditions causing rapid progression of AKI[9-11].

The recognition of risk factors for AKI and treatment aimed at minimising the deleterious effect these risk factors may have on renal function is thus an important part of the initial management of AKI. Assessment of fluid balance, urine output, biochemical derangement and drug therapy are key factors.

Table 5.3 Management of AKI

Management of AKI	Number of patients (%)
Fluid balance chart	518 (88)
TPR chart	515 (87)
Regular monitoring of biochemistry	479 (81)
Catheter	463 (78)
Correction of hypovolaemia	443 (75)
Cessation of nephrotoxic drugs	334 (56)
Non-diuretic drugs administered	195 (33)
Diuretics administered	116 (20)
Central venous pressure	97 (16)
Medications altered to renal doses	91 (15)
Review by renal dietitian or nutrition team	72 (12)
Daily weight chart	56 (9)
Other	51 (9)

Table 5.3 shows what measures were taken to help management in this group of patients. There are some notable facts:

1. Approximately 1 in 5 patients who subsequently died with AKI did not have a urinary catheter inserted.
2. It was not common to alter concomitant drugs dosage in response to AKI. In addition not all patients had nephrotoxic drugs stopped.
3. Review by a renal dietician or nutrition team happened in less than 15% of cases.

This last finding would appear to be in stark contrast to recommendations from the UK Renal Association[12] which state that:

"Referral to a dietician for individual assessment is recommended as nutrient requirements for patients will vary considerably dependent upon the course of the AKI, underlying disease and need for RRT."

Table 5.4 Recording of hourly urine measurements

Hourly urine measurements	Number of patients (%)
Yes	293 (78)
No	81 (22)
Subtotal	374
Not answered	89
Total	463

Whilst bladder catheterisation may not be essential in all cases of AKI, it does enable measurement of hourly urine output and total urine volume. This information can allow early identification of renal impairment. In the 463 patients who did have a urinary catheter inserted there were 81 patients who did not have hourly urine output measurements (Table 5.4). Whilst the reasons behind this omission are probably multifactorial (lack of appreciation of need, lack of appreciation of severity of illness, lack of staff to undertake this, poor recording) it does seem a missed opportunity not to place a catheter in a patient who is developing AKI and not utilise the information fully.

Table 5.5 Adequacy of AKI management

Adequate management of AKI	Number of patients (%)
Yes	375 (71)
No	154 (29)
Subtotal	529
Insufficient data	35
Total	564

The advisors were asked to review the measures taken to manage the patients' AKI and as can be seen from Table 5.5 it was believed that 154/519 patients had inadequacies in clinical management of AKI.

Table 5.6 Omissions in AKI management- advisors' opinion

Omitted from management	Number of patients
Correction of hypovolaemia	85
Biochemistry	62
Fluid	54
Urine output	51
Other	46
Cessation of nephrotoxic drugs	36
Medications altered to Renal doses	32
Urinary Catheter	28
Daily weight chart	23
TPR	21
Central venous pressure	20
Cessation of diuretics	18
Administration of diuretics	15
Review by nutrition team	15
Antibiotics	10
Interventional radiology	3
Total	519

Table 5.6 shows the advisors' reasons for concluding that management of AKI was inadequate for the 154 patients identified in Table 5.5. There were some basic omissions (TPR chart, fluid balance chart, use of a urinary catheter, measurement of urine output on an hourly basis, monitoring of biochemistry), which make it difficult to quantify the degree of physiological derangement and AKI. Without this information it is difficult to see how a sensible management plan can be formulated. NICE has recently made recommendations around the recognition and management of acute illness and state:

"– physiological observations recorded at the time of admission or initial assessment
– a clear written monitoring plan that specifies which physiological observations should be recorded and how often. The plan should take account of the:

> patient's diagnosis
> presence of co-morbidities
> agreed treatment plan." (Appendix 4)

Attention to the recommendations above would ameliorate a substantial portion of the advisors' concerns in this area. Whilst the omissions above reflect poor observational care it was of concern that there were a large number of cases where hypovolaemia was not corrected (85 cases) or nephrotoxic drugs not stopped (36 cases) as these factors will lead to worsening kidney injury.

Table 5.7 Evidence of inappropriate drug usage - Advisors' opinion

Inappropriate drugs used	Number of patients (%)
Yes	52 (9)
No	499 (91)
Subtotal	551
Insufficient data	13
Total	564

Table 5.7 shows data on appropriateness of drug usage in the management of patients recognised with AKI. As can be seen there were 52 patients in whom the advisors believed that problems existed.

Almost half of these cases were concerned with the inappropriate use of diuretics – either administration of diuretics to oliguric, hypovolaemic patients or use of diuretics to try to promote 'polyuric renal failure'. A recent multinational, multicentre, observational study (n = 1,743), evaluated the effect of loop diuretics on clinical outcomes[13]. The study found that although diuretic use was not significantly associated with increased mortality, there was no evidence of benefit either (OR for death was 1.2). There are now several studies showing a lack of effect of diuretics in AKI and based on these data, it is possible to conclude that there is no evidence to support the use of loop diuretics in the prevention of AKI.

Other issues raised by the advisors were around the administration of drugs known to be potential nephrotoxins in the face of deteriorating renal function (aminoglycosides, ACE inhibitors, NSAIDS, contrast media). There needs to be consideration given to the role of these drugs and whether they should be discontinued or the dose modified in the setting of AKI. This may ameliorate further injury to the kidney and was often overlooked in this study.

Finally there were still a few cases of the use of 'renal dose' dopamine despite a wealth of evidence showing no benefit. Three systematic reviews[14-16] and one large RCT[17] evaluating the role of dopamine in preventing deterioration of renal function reached the same conclusion that dopamine did not prevent onset of AKI, need for dialysis, or mortality. Thus, overwhelming evidence exists to suggest that there is no role for "low-dose" dopamine in the prevention of AKI from any aetiology.

Key Findings

178/540 (33%) patients had inadequate investigations. The omissions were basic clinical examination and simple laboratory tests.

63 patients with AKI did not have urinalysis performed.

154/529 (29%) patients had inadequacies in clinical management of AKI. Lack of physiological monitoring was common.

Recognition of acute illness, hypovolaemia and sepsis was poor.

Recommendations

Reagent strip urinalysis should be performed on all emergency admissions. (Clinical Directors and Medical Directors)

NCEPOD recommends that the guidance for recognising the acutely ill patient (NICE CG 50) is disseminated and implemented. In particular all acute patients should have admission physiological observations performed and a written physiological monitoring plan made, taking into account the degree of illness and risk of deterioration. (Clinical Directors and Medical Directors)

Trusts need to put in place a mechanism to ensure that NICE guidance (CG 50) has been implemented. An audit of patients who suffer serious adverse events (cardiac arrest or unplanned admission to critical care) to assess compliance with NICE CG 50 should be presented to the Trust Clinical Governance Committee on an annual basis. (Clinical Directors and Medical Directors)

6 - Referral and support

Often good initial assessment and simple management (adequate volume replacement, treatment of the underlying medical condition (e.g. sepsis, haemorrhage) and avoidance of nephrotoxic medications) will halt deterioration in renal function and allow recovery. However in the event that this does not occur, or there are diagnostic difficulties, further advice and support may be required for optimal patient management.

Table 6.1 Nephrology referrals

Referral to a nephrologist	Number of patients (%)
Yes	181 (32)
No	391 (68)
Subtotal	572
Not answered	20
Total	592

Table 6.1 shows data obtained from the questionnaires completed by the clinicians caring for the patients. From this source 181 patients with AKI were referred to nephrologists for further advice and/or management. The original admitting team, without specialist support, managed the majority of patients (391/572; 68%).

From the casenotes it could be seen that documented nephrology referrals only occurred in 31% (173/561) of cases (Table 6.4).

Time between recognition of AKI and referral to nephrologists (Figure 6.1) revealed that 66% (120/181) were rapidly identified and specialist advice sought. However as can be seen there was quite a large spread of time to referral and in some cases substantial delays were present.

Number of patients

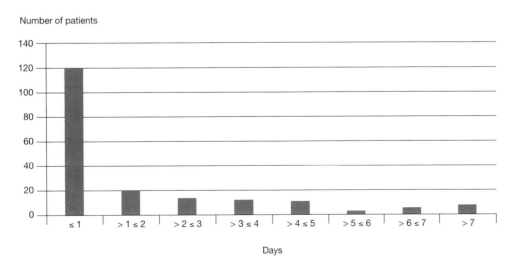

Days

Figure 6.1 Time to nephrology referral from recognition of AKI

Table 6.2 Action following nephrology referral

Level of action	Number of patients
Telephone	78
Ward review	117
Transfer to level 3	28
Transfer to renal unit	30

Table 6.2 shows the outcome of the referral to nephrology. There were multiple answers for 181 patients which makes the data somewhat difficult to interpret. However it was possible to stratify the answers to show the 'highest' level of support that was given as a result of the referral. These data are shown in Table 6.3. One hundred and forty two patients were either reviewed on the ward and/or transferred to a higher level of care. However 38 patients (21% of referrals) were never reviewed by nephrologists and telephone advice was given without patient review. In seven of these 181 cases it was reported that there were difficulties in contacting nephrologists and arranging patient review.

Table 6.3 Highest level of action following nephrology referral

Level of action	Number of patients (%)
Telephone only	38 (21)
Ward review	84 (47)
Transfer to level 2/3	28 (16)
Transfer to renal unit	30 (17)
Subtotal	180
Not answered	1
Total	181

Previous studies in the UK have shown that the majority of AKI is managed by non-specialists. A single centre study from 1997 showed that only 22% of patients with AKI were referred to nephrologists[18]. It does not appear that there have been substantial changes in this practice over the last decade. This underlines the importance of all medical teams having the knowledge and skills to assess and provide good management to patients at risk of and suffering from AKI.

As all patients within this study died it is not clear how decisions about the cause of AKI, appropriateness of treatment or decisions about withholding active treatment of AKI were made. Whilst nephrologists would not wish to be referred every inpatient who developed mild renal impairment or be asked to opine on the utility of renal replacement therapy in patients who were clearly dying' there needs to be some clarity about the role and expectations of nephrology services in our current acute hospital structure.

Table 6.4 Documented nephrology referrals (casenotes)

Evidence of referral to nephrologist	Number of patients (%)
Yes	173 (31)
No	388 (69)
Subtotal	561
Insufficient data	3
Total	564

The National Service Framework for Renal Services recommends that patients at risk of or suffering from AKI should be identified promptly, with hospital services delivering high-quality, clinically appropriate care in partnership with specialised renal teams[19]. Different models of care will be determined by local resource availability and geography but there are essentially three different in-patient venues – the critical care unit, the renal unit and the non-specialist ward. Interaction between different disciplines is important to ensure correct initial placement of the patient and appropriate subsequent care.

Referrals are often hampered by a complex set of delays involving both the recognition of AKI and acting on that recognition. There is a large group of AKI patients with moderate renal impairment, in whom timely intervention may abort progression to a more severe degree of AKI. Such early intervention has the potential to reduce the morbidity and mortality of this condition. Table 6.5 shows the advisors' opinions as to the timeliness of referral.

**Table 6.5 Timeliness of nephrology referral –
advisors' opinion**

Was referral timely	Number of patients (%)
Yes	132 (79)
No	35 (21)
Subtotal	167
Insufficient data	6
Total	173

Of the 167 cases that could be assessed, 35 patients were not referred to a nephrologist in a timely manner in the opinion of the advisors. The advisors commented that there were often long delays between the recognition of AKI and subsequent referral for advice and support. The reasons for these delays were not clear; it may have related to lack of appreciation of the seriousness of AKI or may reflect that the referring team were putting in place simple measures to treat the AKI that did not require specialist advice.

The majority of the referrals for nephrology support were considered appropriate by the advisors; in only nine cases was it considered to be inappropriate.

**Table 6.6 Appropriateness of nephrology advice –
Advisors' opinion**

Appropriate advice	Number of patients (%)
Yes	135 (84)
No	26 (16)
Subtotal	161
Insufficient data	12
Total	173

The advice given by nephrology was considered to be appropriate in 135/161 cases. In those 26 cases where advisors had concerns about the advice given, the major issues seem to have been lack of appreciation of severity of illness and assessment of volaemic status (Table 6.6).

**Table 6.7 Adequacy of nephrology reviews –
Advisors' opinion**

Frequency of reviews adequate	Number of patients (%)
Yes	141 (88)
No	20 (12)
Subtotal	161
Insufficient data	12
Total	173

Of the 173 patients who were referred to a nephrologist, the majority had adequate communication with the renal team after the initial referral. In 20/161 cases the advisors were of the opinion that more frequent input from the renal team was required (Table 6.7).

Case study 7

An elderly patient presented with a one week history of vomiting and confusion. Initial blood tests revealed urea 34mmol/l, creatinine 1160micromol/l and potassium 6.9mmol/l. Resuscitation was commenced with fluid, dextrose/insulin and sodium bicarbonate. Urgent renal ultrasound ruled out urinary obstruction. The patient was referred for nephrology advice. The nephrology SpR gave telephone advice only; this consisted of continuing with the resuscitation plan and repeat assessment of U&Es in a few hours. The nephrology SpR was contacted 6 hours later as the potassium was 6.6mmol/l. Telephone advice at that time was to keep well hydrated, perform a vasculitic screen and ring back again if hyperkalaemia persisted. The patient had a cardiac arrest some hours later. Potassium at the time of cardiac arrest was 7.7mmol/l.

The advisors considered that the advice given by the nephrology SpR did not help in patient management and that earlier transfer to a nephrology unit should have occurred.

Perhaps more of an issue than the delayed referrals were the group of patients who never had specialist advice. As can be seen from table 6.8 the advisors considered that of the 388 patients who were not referred to a nephrologist, 77 should have been referred for advice and support (20%).

Table 6.8 Need for nephrology referral in the group of patients not referred – Advisors' opinion

Patient should have been referred	Number of patients (%)
Yes	77 (20)
No	302 (80)
Subtotal	379
Insufficient data	9
Total	388

Table 6.9 Reason referral required – Advisors' opinion

Reason referral necessary	Number of patients
Clinical opinion	44
Management without RRT	23
RRT	4
Other	3
Subtotal	74
Not answered	3
Total	77

From Table 6.9 it can be seen that in the majority of cases the referral should have been for an expert clinical opinion (44 cases) or for management advice, excluding RRT (23 cases).

Taken together these data show that in this study there were deficiencies in the initial assessment and management of patients with AKI; that less than one third of patients with AKI were referred to nephrologists and that there are often delays in making the referral. This is not in keeping with the National Service Framework for Renal Services[19] which states:

"QUALITY REQUIREMENT THREE: People at risk of, or suffering from, acute renal failure are identified promptly, with hospital services delivering high quality, clinically appropriate care in partnership with specialised renal teams.
Markers of good practice
• Timely identification and referral to renal and critical care services for specialist, culturally appropriate advice and assessment."

* Acute renal failure is now termed acute kidney injury.

There was no difference in the advisors' opinion of the quality of care irrespective of nephrology referral (Table 6.10).

However, when the patients who were referred in a timely manner and received an appropriate response from nephrology services were isolated the picture was quite different (Table 6.11). In this group the advisors judged that there was a much higher percentage of good practice (slightly over two thirds).

Table 6.10 Overall quality of care and nephrology referral

	Referred to nephrologist	Not referred to nephrologist
Overall assessment of care - advisors' opinion	Number of patients (%)	Number of patients (%)
Good practice	92 (54)	188 (49)
Room for improvement - clinical	45 (26)	130 (34)
Room for improvement - organisational	5 (3)	11 (3)
Room for improvement - clinical & organisational	17 (10)	26 (7)
Less than satisfactory	11 (6)	31 (8)
Total	**170**	**386**

Table 6.11 Overall quality of care and timely nephrology referral with correct advice

	Timely referral and correct advice
Overall assessment of care - advisors' opinion	Number of patients (%)
Good practice	77 (69)
Room for improvement - clinical	20 (18)
Room for improvement - organisational	5 (5)
Room for improvement - clinical & organisational	5 (5)
Less than satisfactory	4 (4)
Total	**111**

6 - REFERRAL AND SUPPORT

Key Findings

173/561 (31%) patients were referred to a nephrologist for advice or management support.

35/167 (21%) referrals to nephrology were considered by the advisors to be delayed.

77/379 (20%) patients who were not referred to a nephrologist, should have been referred for advice and support in the view of the advisors.

The advisors judged quality of care to be good in 69% of patients who were referred to nephrologists in a timely manner and in whom the advice given was appropriate (111 patients).

Recommendations

When referral is made for specialist advice from nephrologists prompt senior advice and a review where appropriate is required. All patients with AKI should be promptly discussed by the renal registrar with their consultants. (Clinical Directors and Medical Directors)

Every hospital should have a written guideline detailing how the three clinical areas where patients with AKI are treated (critical care unit, the renal unit and the non-specialist ward) interact to ensure delivery of high quality, clinically appropriate care for patients with AKI. (Clinical Directors and Medical Directors)

7 - Renal replacement therapy

Patients who develop AKI and have complications of electrolyte imbalance (particularly hyperkalaemia), acidosis and volume overload are likely to die unless renal support is provided. In the acute context this is usually intermittent haemodialysis or a continuous haemofiltration technique. Both of these can be termed renal replacement therapy (RRT).

Table 7.1 Documented evidence of RRT

RRT administered	Number of patients (%)
Yes	67 (12)
No	484 (88)
Subtotal	**551**
Insufficient data	13
Total	**564**

Sixty seven patients had RRT delivered to them. This represents 67/551 (12%) of patients in this study (Table 7.1).

Table 7.2 Type of RRT administered

Type of RRT	Number of patients
Intermittent	32
Continuous	35
Total	**67**

There was a fairly equal mix of continuous and intermittent techniques of RRT used (Table 7.2). The advisors agreed that the type of RRT used was appropriate in all but three cases. These were three cases where it was judged that intermittent RRT was not appropriate and that a continuous technique should have been used.

It may appear remarkable that such a low percentage of patients who died due to AKI received RRT. However, it must be remembered that often AKI is a reflection of multi-system disease and that RRT may not alter the eventual outcome.

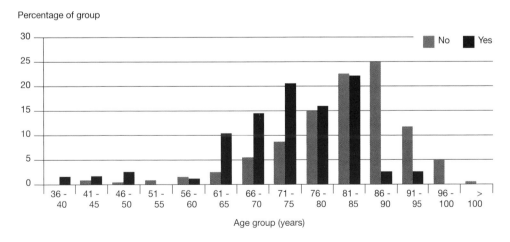

Figure 7.1 Age distribution and administration of RRT

Figure 7.1 shows the age distribution of patients broken down by whether or not RRT was delivered. Those patients who did not have RRT had a median age of 84 years (range 41-102); those patients who did have RRT delivered had a median age of 75 years (range 39-91). Overall, within the study there was an equal sex distribution. However when analysed by whether RRT was delivered there was a slight difference (RRT delivered – 56% male, 44% female; RRT not delivered – 48% male, 52% female).

It has previously been shown that elderly patients are less likely to be referred to nephrologists[20-21] and it does appear that RRT was delivered less frequently to older patients in this study. This may be a reflection of underlying disease and lack of reversibility. However, it must be remembered that chronological age and physiological age are not identical and age itself should not be used to limit access to therapy or treatment.

There may be differences in perception between physicians (general and care of the elderly) and nephrologists[22]. This study revealed that more patients would have been accepted for RRT by nephrologists than would have been referred by general and care of the elderly physicians and concluded that there may be under-referral of elderly patients with renal failure to nephrologists. A major challenge is to ensure proper team working and communication between specialties to ensure that patients are optimally managed.

Table 7.3 shows overall quality of care broken down by use of RRT. It appears that there are substantial differences between these two groups with a higher proportion of patients judged to have received good care in the group that had RRT (69% v 47%).

Twenty nine patients received RRT in a renal unit and 38 received RRT in a critical care unit.

Of the 29 patients receiving RRT in a renal unit 26 underwent an intermittent technique. Of the 38 patients receiving RRT in a critical care unit only six patients underwent an intermittent technique with the remaining 32 undergoing continuous haemofiltration.

Table 7.3 Overall quality of care and RRT administration

	No evidence of RRT	Evidence of RRT
Advisors' opinion on overall care	Number of patients (%)	Number of patients (%)
Good practice	226 (47)	46 (69)
Room for improvement - clinical	164 (34)	9 (13)
Room for improvement - organisational	15 (3)	1 (1)
Room for improvement - clinical & organisational	36 (8)	7 (10)
Less than satisfactory	38 (8)	4 (6)
Total	479	67

There were clear differences in practice depending on where RRT was delivered. Intermittent haemodialysis was more likely to be performed in a renal unit where as continuous haemofiltration was more likely to be used in a critical care unit. These differences are likely to be based on custom and practice and familiarity/availability of equipment rather than evidence based. The most recent evidence suggests that intermittent haemodialysis and continuous RRT appear to lead to similar clinical outcomes for patients with AKI[23-24].

There was evidence in the casenotes that 74 patients were transferred to a critical care unit (level 2 or level 3 care) during their inpatient stay. Of these patients, 33 received RRT.

Table 7.4 Documented renal team input on critical care wards

Documented input from renal team	Number of patients (%)
Yes	25 (40)
No	37 (60)
Subtotal	**62**
Insufficient data	12
Total	**74**

Only 25 patients out of 62 had documented input from the renal team during their critical care stay (Table 7.4). It was believed that in three of these 25 cases the input from nephrology was inadequate. Clearly provision of RRT is a core service within critical care units and that alone does not mandate input from the renal team (in the same way that the requirement for ventilation or inotropic support does not mandate input of respiratory physicians or cardiologists). However in cases of diagnostic difficulty or to enable smooth transition of patient care both before and after critical care then involvement of renal services is essential. There should be clear guidelines detailing the role of renal services within critical care to ensure optimum patient management and continuity of care.

Table 7.5 Patients that would have benefited from RRT – Advisors' opinion

RRT required	Number of patients (%)
Yes	36 (8)
No	391 (92)
Subtotal	**427**
Insufficient data	57
Total	**484**

Table 7.4 shows the advisors opinion in those patients who did not receive RRT. Out of 427 patients the advisors believed that 36 should have received RRT as part of their treatment plan.

In five cases there was intent to provide RRT but the patients died prior to initiation of therapy. In three cases there was lack of an immediately available critical care bed to provide support. These eight cases perhaps underline the pressure that critical care/renal services are under at present. In several other cases it was felt that more aggressive treatment including RRT should have been provided as patient outcome was uncertain.

Case study 8

An elderly patient was admitted to hospital with non-specific deterioration and was found to have AKI on admission (urea 37mmol/l, creatinine 550micromol/l). The cause was felt to be multifactorial (Type II diabetes, ischaemic heart disease, NSAIDS, diuretics and an acute diarrhoeal illness). Despite volume replacement and cessation of nephrotoxic drugs renal function did not recover and a decision was made not to institute renal replacement therapy. There was no record of discussion about renal replacement therapy with either the patient or next of kin in the notes.

The advisors felt that this patient, although elderly, was independent and mobile and had reversible AKI. In view of this it was felt that renal replacement therapy should have been instituted.

Case study 9

An elderly patient developed AKI after admission to hospital. In view of oliguria, hyperkalaemia and acidosis a nephrology opinion was sought. The patient was reviewed promptly by an SpR in nephrology. At the time of review the blood pressure was recorded as 95/50. A previous echocardiogram showed mild left ventricular dysfunction. The nephrology SpR provided some advice on fluid management but concluded that due to left ventricular dysfunction the patient was not a candidate for renal replacement therapy. It did not appear that there was any consultant oversight of this decision. The patient died 48 hours later.

The advisors felt that this patient should have been offered renal replacement therapy and that there were no significant co-morbidities that precluded this. Furthermore the advisors were concerned that an SpR, without consultant oversight, was making treatment limitation decisions.

Table 7.6 Overall quality of care and the need for RRT

	No	Yes
Advisors' opinion on overall care	Number of patients (%)	Number of patients (%)
Good practice	203 (52)	1 (3)
Room for improvement - clinical	130 (34)	15 (42)
Room for improvement - organisational	10 (3)	4 (11)
Room for improvement - clinical & organisational	20 (5)	5 (14)
Less than satisfactory	24 (6)	11 (31)
Total	**387**	**36**

Table 7.6 shows the advisors' opinion of quality of overall care in those patients who did not receive RRT, broken down by advisor opinion of whether this was the correct decision or not. There were 36 patients who did not receive RRT but it was believed they should have received RRT. The quality of care was judged to be low and almost one third judged as less than satisfactory.

Decision to withdraw or not to treat AKI

As stated previously the development of AKI may be judged to be a terminal event and a consequence of severe illness rather than a major contributory factor in the dying process. Under these conditions, a decision may be made either to withdraw remedial AKI treatment that has already been initiated or, not to initiate treatment at all (much in the same way that a decision is made not to attempt cardiopulmonary resuscitation in some patients who suffer a cardiac arrest). Only 67 patients within this study had RRT and it would therefore appear that treatment limitation decisions were being made. In 308/592 (52%) of cases the clinician indicated that a decision was made not to treat, or to withdraw from treating the AKI. Table 7.7 shows those who were involved in the decision making process.

The consultant in charge was not involved in decision making about treatment limitation in 23 cases (7%). Whilst it is possible that there was consultant input from either nephrology or critical care in these cases it surely should be expected that the consultant in charge should be involved at all times.

It appears that there was quite low patient involvement in the decision making process about treatment limitation. This may reflect a reluctance to discuss death and dying with patients or may be that these very sick patients were judged not to be competent to take part in this process. Earlier involvement of patients in decisions about their treatment, prior to clinical deterioration, may solve the latter problem. The GMC provides good guidance on treatment limitation decisions[25] and these must be applied to our patients. The Mental Capacity Act[26] sets out the legislative framework with regards to capacity of patients to take part in decisions about treatment options. It also makes clear the responsibilities of doctors to assess capacity and where capacity is lacking to consult with close family or friends. In the absence of any close family or friends it is the responsibility of each Trust to have formal arrangements for dealing with this (usually in the form of an Independent Mental Capacity Advocate)[26].

Table 7.7 Those involved in the decision to withdraw from, or not to initiate treatment of, AKI

Consultant in charge	285
Renal team	73
Critical care	72
Patient	56
Relatives	216

Case study 10

An elderly patient was admitted to hospital as an emergency due to a chest infection. Significant co-morbidities existed (type II diabetes, ischaemic heart disease, previous myocardial infarction, left ventricular failure, chronic kidney disease, chronic obstructive pulmonary disease, morbid obesity). Renal function deteriorated despite good medical care. Advice was requested from a consultant nephrologist who discussed treatment options with the patient and next of kin. After several discussions, the patient decided that they did not want to undergo renal replacement therapy.

Advisors commented that early recognition of deterioration allowed the patient to take part in decision making about treatment options. Furthermore open discussions about the likely outcome, in view of multiple and severe co-morbidities, helped the patient understand the likely eventual outcome. Advisors commented that this was excellent care of a dying patient.

Case study 11

An elderly patient was admitted from home following severe vomiting and diarrhoea. They had significant cardiorespiratory co-morbidity but was self caring and able to live independently with their spouse. On admission a diagnosis of AKI secondary to volume depletion was made. Despite resuscitation the biochemistry did not improve and no urine was passed. There was no discussion with the patient about likely outcomes and appropriate treatments. Over the next 24 hours the patient became more drowsy and hypotensive. A decision not to escalate care was taken following discussion with their spouse and a palliative care plan put in place. On that day an ultrasound (that had been requested on admission) revealed bilateral hydronephroses. The patient died later that day.

The advisors were concerned that the decision not to escalate care had been made without a full assessment and that hydronephrosis was an easily reversible cause of AKI. Furthermore, no effort had been made to discuss treatment options with the patient when they were competent.

Advisors were asked about the appropriateness of treatment limitation decisions. In 18 cases they judged that this decision was made without all relevant clinical opinions being taken into account whilst in 290 cases clinical input was judged to be good. It was believed that the decision to limit treatment was appropriate in 284 cases but inappropriate in 17 cases.

Key Findings

Only 67/551 (12%) patients received RRT.

Of the 427 patients who did not receive RRT the advisors judged that 36 (8%) should have received RRT as part of their treatment plan.

Older patients received less RRT in this study. Above the age of 85 very few patients received RRT.

Treatment limitations were made in 52% of patients in this study. Patient involvement was low.

Recommendations

Early recognition of at risk patients should allow patient involvement in treatment limitation decisions before clinical condition deteriorates and the opportunity for this involvement is missed. (Clinical Directors and Medical Directors)

Treatment limitation decisions should be made with reference to guidance produced by the GMC and within the legislative framework of the Mental Capacity Act. (Clinical Directors and Medical Directors)

8 - Recognition of severity of illness

It is well known that failure to recognise severity of illness in hospitalised patients is common and that there is often a failure to act even when recognition has occurred[27-31].

Table 8.1 Adequacy of senior reviews – advisors' opinion

Adequate senior reviews	Number of patients (%)
Yes	415 (76)
No	134 (24)
Subtotal	549
Insufficient data	15
Total	564

The advisors judged that quality of care in those cases with inadequate senior reviews was less good. Whilst this is merely an association it does highlight the importance that the advisors placed on adequacy of senior review. It is also intuitive that good care is more likely to be associated with sufficiently senior doctors seeing the patients regularly.

NICE have recently published a clinical guideline for the recognition and assessment of the acutely unwell inpatient (Appendix 4). This comprehensive document takes note of previous NCEPOD work[8] and makes recommendations to provide a structure for recognising and responding to acute illness. One of the major elements of these recommendations is a track and

Table 8.2 Overall quality of care and adequacy of senior reviews

Advisors' opinion on overall care	Adequate senior reviews Number of patients (%)	Inadequate senior reviews Number of patients (%)
Good practice	260 (63)	12 (9)
Room for improvement - clinical	119 (29)	55 (41)
Room for improvement - organisational	12 (3)	4 (3)
Room for improvement - clinical & organisational	14 (3)	28 (21)
Less than satisfactory	8 (2)	35 (26)
Total	413	134

A regular and senior medical review of these sick patients is one component of early recognition and successful management. Table 8.1 shows that 134 patients, in the opinion of the advisors, did not have adequate senior reviews. The overall quality of care in the two groups (adequate/inadequate senior reviews) is in Table 8.2.

trigger system. This consists of an appropriate monitoring tool which can track changes in patient condition (e.g. MEWS) to ensure rapid identification of these high risk patients and a structure to ensure an appropriate response (Appendix 5). Part of the appropriate response suggested by NICE is the use of outreach teams to support ward staff and ensure timely treatment and transfer if appropriate.

Table 8.3 Documented involvement of outreach

Evidence of outreach involvement	Number of patients (%)
Yes	79 (15)
No	458 (85)
Subtotal	537
Insufficient data	27
Total	564

Table 8.3 shows that in this group of patients who all died, there was involvement of outreach services in only 79 cases (15%).

Table 8.4 Patients who would have benefited from outreach input – Advisors' opinion

Outreach involvement would have been beneficial	Number of patients (%)
Yes	106 (24)
No	331 (76)
Subtotal	437
Insufficient data	21
Total	458

In the opinion of the advisors an additional 106 patients would have potentially benefited from involvement of outreach services (Table 8.4). It is worth noting that the advisors stated that 331 patients who were never referred to outreach would not have benefited from their involvement. Given that these patients all subsequently died it may be that the advisors felt this outcome was inevitable and no further advice could be useful or it may be that there is some scepticism about the role of outreach amongst this group of physicians.

In order to receive an appropriate level of care patients often require transfer to a renal or critical care unit. If RRT is required then this is usually delivered following transfer to an appropriate unit. However many patients with renal failure who do not require RRT are very sick and would also benefit from expert management in a renal or critical care unit.

Table 8.5 Documented patient transfers

Transferred	Number of patients
Renal unit	39
Level 3	50
Level 2	24
Other	14
Subtotal	127
Not transferred	311
Not answered	126
Total	564

Table 8.5 shows that 113 patients were transferred to a renal or critical care unit whilst 311 patients were not transferred. It is a reflection of the quality of note keeping that it was impossible to answer this question in 126/564 cases (22%). NCEPOD has previously commented on the quality of note keeping and it is disappointing that little seems to have changed over many years in this respect.

Table 8.6 Patients who would have benefited from a transfer to critical care – Advisors' opinion

Patient should have been transferred	Number of patients (%)
Yes	44 (16)
No	229 (84)
Subtotal	273
Insufficient data	38
Total	311

Of the 273 patients who were not transferred the advisors stated that 44 patients should have been transferred to a higher level of care.

Table 8.7 Reason transfer to critical care was required – Advisors' opinion

Reason transfer required	Number of patients
More acute care	41
RRT	9
Cardio-respiratory support	2
Other	2

Table 8.8 shows data on advisors' opinion of overall quality of care in those patients transferred to a critical care or renal unit compared to those who were not transferred. It appears that the group who were transferred to a higher level of care were judged to have received better care than those who were not, the difference being better clinical care.

Patients not transferred to renal/critical care unit split by correct decision (no) vs incorrect decision (yes).

Table 8.8 Overall quality of care and transfer to critical care or renal unit

	Not transferred	Transferred
Advisors' opinion on overall care	Number of patients (%)	Number of patients (%)
Good practice	142 (46)	67 (60)
Room for improvement - clinical	110 (36)	23 (21)
Room for improvement - organisational	9 (3)	1 (1)
Room for improvement - clinical & organisational	26 (8)	12 (11)
Less than satisfactory	21 (7)	9 (8)
Total	**308**	**112**

The reasons that advisors considered transfer should have taken place are given in Table 8.7 (answers may be multiple for each patient). As stated at the beginning of this section, these patients are often very sick and require a higher level of care than can be given on a general ward. This was reflected in the fact that in the opinion of the advisors only 9/44 patients required a transfer for RRT with the majority requiring more acute care and support (excluding RRT).

Table 8.9 Overall quality of care of patients that required a transfer to critical care or a renal unit

	Required transfer to critical care	
	No	Yes
Advisors' opinion on overall care	Number of patients (%)	Number of patients (%)
Good practice	120 (53)	1 (2)
Room for improvement - clinical	83 (36)	16 (36)
Room for improvement - organisational	6 (3)	1 (2)
Room for improvement - clinical & organisational	9 (4)	16 (36)
Less than satisfactory	10 (4)	10 (23)
Total	**228**	**44**

Table 8.9 shows data on patients who were not transferred to a critical care or renal unit. There were more striking differences when the advisor opinion about quality of care were examined in those patients in whom they believed transfer would have been appropriate but never happened: in this group there was judged to be substantial room for improvement and less than satisfactory care.

8 - RECOGNITION OF SEVERITY OF ILLNESS

Key Findings

134/549 patients did not have adequate senior reviews. These patients were judged by the advisors to have less good care overall.

Critical care outreach services were involved in 79/537 cases. It was believed, by the advisors, that they should have been involved in a further 106 cases.

113 patients were transferred to renal/critical care. The advisors were of the view that an additional 44 should have received step up care.

Patients who did not receive appropriate step up care were judged by the advisors to have an overall quality of care that was poor.

Recommendations

All acute admissions should receive adequate senior reviews (with a consultant review within 12 hours of admission as previously recommended by NCEPOD[3]. (Clinical Directors and Medical Directors)

There should be sufficient critical care and renal beds to allow rapid step up in care if appropriate. (Department of Health)

63

9 - Organisation of renal services

The quality of care delivered to patients with AKI will be dependent on the facilities available within each hospital. Not all hospitals have facilities for renal replacement therapy, access to specialist nephrology advice or renal units providing dialysis. Furthermore the care of patients with renal disease is reliant upon renal support services other than medical staff such as dieticians and pharmacists. In order to gauge the prevalence of renal facilities, NCEPOD sent an Organisational Questionnaire to a contact in each hospital asking specifically about resources available.

Table 9.1 Ability to admit acute emergency admissions

Acute emergency admissions	Number of hospitals (%)
Yes	221 (72)
No	84 (28)
Total	**305**

The number of hospitals that accepted emergency admissions was found to be 221/305 (Table 9.1).

Table 9.2 Onsite nephrologists and ability to admit acute emergency admissions

	Hospital accepts acute emergency admissions		
	Yes	No	Total
Onsite nephrologists	Number of hospitals (%)	Number of hospitals (%)	Number of hospitals (%)
Yes	99 (46)	6 (7)	105 (35)
No	118 (54)	78 (93)	196 (65)
Subtotal	**217**	**84**	**301**
Not answered	4	0	4
Total	**221**	**84**	**305**

Table 9.3 Type of nephrologists

Onsite nephrologists	Number of hospitals
Specialist nephrologists	92
General physician with specialist interest	9
Subtotal	**101**
Not answered	4
Total	**105**

The number of hospitals that had nephrologists onsite was 105/301 (35%) of which 92/101 (91%) had specialist nephrologists, whilst 9/101 (9%) had physicians with a specialist interest in nephrology. Of the hospitals accepting acute admissions, only 99/217 (46%) hospitals had onsite nephrologists. AKI affects up to 20% of hospitalised patients and insufficient nephrology presence may alter of these patients. Thus it can be seen that acute admitting hospitals lack the requisite complement of trained nephrologists to respond to the under recognised morbidity presented by AKI.

For those hospitals that did not have onsite nephrologists, NCEPOD asked where the nearest nephrologists were based. Table 9.4 shows the result of this analysis.

Table 9.4 Proximity of nearest nephrologists for hospitals without in-house service

Nearest nephrologist	Number of hospitals (%)
Same trust	59 (38)
Same city different trust	35 (23)
Different city	61 (39)
Subtotal	155
Not answered	41
Total	196

As shown in Table 9.4, for 35/155 (23%) hospitals without onsite nephrologists the nearest nephrologist was in the same city but a different Trust and in 61/155 (39%) hospitals without onsite nephrologists, the nearest nephrologists were in a different city.

Furthermore, NCEPOD also enquired whether each hospital had access to on call nephrological advice (in-house or otherwise) (Table 9.5). It was found that 42/298 did not have access; of these, only six had a referral protocol for such advice. NCEPOD believes that as an ideal, all acute admitting Trusts should have onsite nephrologists; but where that is logistically difficult, nephrological advice should be available within the same city. Moreover all hospitals, acute or otherwise, should be able to access nephrological advice when needed and there should be a clear referral protocol for access to such advice. It is perhaps fair to surmise that the incidence of AKI related mortality will not be reduced unless there is a re-organisation of access to renal teams.

Table 9.5 Access to on call nephrologists

	Hospital accepts acute emergency admissions		
	Yes	No	Total
Access to on call nephrologists	Number of hospitals (%)	Number of hospitals (%)	Number of hospitals (%)
Yes	204 (94)	52 (64)	256 (86)
No	13 (6)	29 (36)	42 (14)
Subtotal	217	81	298
Not answered	4	3	7
Total	221	84	305

Table 9.6 Renal units

| Renal unit onsite | Hospital accepts acute emergency admissions | | |
| | Yes | No | Total |
	Number of hospitals (%)	Number of hospitals (%)	Number of hospitals (%)
Yes	113 (52)	8 (10)	121 (40)
No	103 (48)	76 (90)	179 (60)
Subtotal	216	84	300
Not answered	5	0	5
Total	221	84	305

Table 9.7 Type of renal unit

| Type of renal unit | Hospital accepts acute emergency admissions | | |
| | Yes | No | Total |
	Number of hospitals (%)	Number of hospitals (%)	Number of hospitals (%)
Main dialysing	55 (49)	1 (13)	56 (47)
Satellite	57 (51)	7 (87)	64 (53)
Subtotal	112	8	120
Not answered	1	0	1
Total	113	8	121

Dedicated renal units have an important part to play in the management of AKI; not only as foci of expert opinion but also as a dedicated area for the administration of renal replacement therapy. The data shows that 121/300 (40%) hospitals had a renal unit (Table 9.6); of which 56/120 were main dialysing units and 64/120 satellite units (one site did not define themselves) (Table 9.7).

Of the 179/300 (60%) hospitals without a renal unit 77/155 had formal access to a unit with 76/155 accessing it as a tertiary referral centre (Table 9.8). It should be noted that 24/179 hospitals did not answer this question. One would hope that the specific details of access to renal units were unknown to the respondent rather than there being no access available.

Table 9.8 Links with renal units

Links with renal unit	Number of hospitals (%)
Formal link	77 (50)
Tertiary referral	76 (50)
Subtotal	155
Not answered	24
Total	179

Renal replacement therapy can be administered in locations other than renal units. It is possible for forms of haemodialysis to be administered in settings such as level 3 and level 2 units. NCEPOD enquired about the availability of RRT in these areas. The proportion of hospitals with level 2/3 units is shown in Table 9.9; and the proportion of these that can deliver RRT is shown in Table 9.10.

Table 9.9 Availability of level 2/3 units

| | Hospital accepts acute emergency admissions | | |
| | Yes | No | Total |
Critical care wards	Number of hospitals (%)	Number of hospitals (%)	Number of hospitals (%)
Level 2 and 3	172 (83)	3 (9)	175 (72)
Level 3	19 (9)	1 (3)	20 (8)
Level 2	17 (8)	31 (89)	48 (20)
Subtotal	**208**	**35**	**243**
Neither	13	49	62
Total	**221**	**84**	**305**

Table 9.10 Ability to deliver RRT in level 2/3 setting

| | RRT administered | | | | | |
Type of units	Level 2 and 3	Level 3	Level 2	Subtotal	Neither	Total
Level 2 and 3	75	80	0	155	20	**175**
Level 3	-	14	-	14	6	**20**
Level 2	-	-	1	1	47	**48**
Total	**75**	**94**	**1**	**170**	**73**	**243**

From the organisational questionnaire 169/195 (87%) hospitals which had level 3 beds could deliver RRT on these units. This was further analysed to look at the ability to deliver RRT in level 2 beds, the percentage able to administer RRT fell to 76/223 (34%). It is of note that 13% of units providing level 3 care could not deliver RRT. This could be due to respondent units not classifying haemofiltration as RRT.

Table 9.11 RRT prescriptions on level 2 and level 3

Who prescribes RRT	Number of hospitals (%)
Intensivists	98 (58)
Nephrologists	16 (9)
Intensivists/nephrologists	54 (32)
Intensivists/nephrologists/other	1 (<1)
Intensivists/other	1 (<1)
Total	170

Of the level 2/3 units that did provide RRT, greater than 50% was prescribed by the intensivist with only 16/170 being prescribed by nephrologists alone (Table 9.11). There was evidence of joint management with 37/170 hospitals taking a combined approach to the prescription of RRT. Where appropriate, nephrologists should be more closely involved in managing patients receiving RRT on level 2/3 units in order to maximise specialist input. This is most important when a patient has AKI which is either resistant or has an unusual aetiology.

Table 9.12 Access to out of hours ultrasound (US) (weekdays)

	Hospital accepts acute emergency admissions		
	Yes	No	Total
Urgent US weekdays out of hours	Number of hospitals (%)	Number of hospitals (%)	Number of hospitals (%)
Yes	192 (88)	48 (58)	240 (80)
No	26 (12)	35 (42)	61 (20)
Subtotal	218	83	301
Not answered	3	1	4
Total	221	84	305

Table 9.13 Access to ultrasound (weekends)

	Hospital accepts acute emergency admissions		
	Yes	No	Total
Urgent US weekend	Number of hospitals (%)	Number of hospitals (%)	Number of hospitals (%)
Yes	190 (87)	42 (53)	232 (78)
No	28 (13)	38 (47)	66 (22)
Subtotal	218	80	298
Not answered	3	4	7
Total	221	84	305

Table 9.14 Access to out of hours nephrostomy insertion (weekdays)

	Hospital accepts acute emergency admissions		
	Yes	No	Total
Urgent nephrostomy weekdays out of hours	Number of hospitals (%)	Number of hospitals (%)	Number of hospitals (%)
Yes	151 (70)	26 (32)	177 (60)
No	65 (30)	55 (68)	120 (40)
Subtotal	216	81	297
Not answered	5	5	8
Total	221	86	305

Table 9.15 Access to nephrostomy insertion (weekends)

	Hospital accepts acute emergency admissions		
	Yes	No	Total
Urgent nephrostomy weekend	Number of hospitals (%)	Number of hospitals (%)	Number of hospitals (%)
Yes	145 (68)	25 (32)	170 (58)
No	67 (32)	54 (68)	121 (42)
Subtotal	212	79	291
Not answered	9	5	14
Total	221	84	305

Good care of patients with AKI is dependant upon adequate radiology services. Renal imaging gives important diagnostic information, whilst interventional radiology is of particular importance in the management of obstructive uropathy; nephrostomy being the primary salvage procedure. Thus access to renal ultrasound and the ability to insert a nephrostomy are vital services and ideally should be available 24 hours a day, 7 days per week. This study shows that 240/301 (80%) hospitals had access to renal ultrasound out of hours and 232/298 (78%) at the weekend (Tables 9.12 and 9.13). In addition, it was only possible to arrange nephrostomy insertion in

Case study 12

An elderly patient was admitted with general deterioration and found to be in acute on chronic kidney disease. An ultrasound scan was requested, but despite this and evidence of deteriorating renal function, this was not performed until four days post-admission. The scan revealed bilateral hydronephroses. Consequently, the urologists advised urgent bilateral nephrostomy insertion which was undertaken radiologically that day.

The advisors were concerned about the delay in arranging an ultrasound of the renal tract considering the eventual requirement for bilateral nephrostomies, and felt this case illustrated the necessity for urgent access to renal imaging services.

Case study 13

A patient was admitted with recurrent hypoglycaemic episodes and found to be in renal failure with anuria and metabolic acidosis. Despite regular clinical review an ultrasound of the kidneys was not arranged until three days post-admission; this showed an absent right kidney and obstruction of the single left kidney. The following day an urgent nephrostomy was arranged with good drainage. A subsequent CT scan showed the cause of obstruction to be a single calculus in the distal ureter.

Advisors were concerned that there should be such a delay in renal imaging of an anuric patient especially when the cause of the AKI was eminently treatable.

177/297 (60%) of hospitals out of hours and 170/291 (58%) at the weekend (Tables 9.14 and 9.15). AKI is often an emergency presentationand it is axiomatic that emergency admissions can present at any time of the day or day of the week (as the study data shows); thus modalities to investigate and treat AKI must be available at all the times. This is perhaps most important in obstructive uropathy where early drainage of blocked urinary outflow will improve the prognosis for recovering renal function. It was a recurrent theme amongst the advisors that there was evidence of delayed radiology. Case studies 12 and 13 illustrate the importance of timely nephrostomy insertion.

This study also reviewed where renal biopsies were reported and found that 113/270 were reported within the same hospital with 150/270 being sent to a specialist site (Table 9.16). Seven hospitals indicated that renal biopsies were reported in their own laboratory and a specialist centre.

Table 9.16 Site of biopsy reporting

	Hospital accepts acute emergency admissions		
	Yes	No	Total
Renal biopsies	Number of hospitals (%)	Number of hospitals (%)	Number of hospitals (%)
Own pathology lab	97 (47)	16 (25)	113 (42)
Specialist centre	104 (50)	46 (73)	150 (56)
Both	6 (3)	1 (2)	7 (3)
Subtotal	207	63	270
Not answered	14	21	35
Total	221	84	305

The availability and prevalence of renal dieticians, renal pharmacists and renal nutrition teams within each hospital was can be seen in Table 9.17.

Table 9.17 Availability of support services

	Renal unit		
Renal support services	Yes	No	Total
Dietician, nutrition team & pharmacist	27	3	30
Dietician	19	5	24
Dietician & nutrition team	2	1	3
Dietician & pharmacist	28	1	29
Pharmacist	0	3	3
Subtotal	76	13	89
No support services	45	166	211
Total	121	179	300

Five hospitals did not say if they had a renal unit onsite

Table 9.17 shows that 211/300 (70%) hospitals did not have any of these renal support services. That such a high proportion of hospitals purport to have no access to such services is remarkable. It would be desirable that all hospitals had both dieticians and pharmacists who although not renal-dedicated had knowledge and/or experience in AKI which could be utilised as required.

Key Findings

More than half of acute admitting hospitals did not have onsite nephrologists (118/217: 54%).

For 61/155 (39%) of all hospitals without nephrologists, the nearest nephrologist was in a different city.

Not all hospitals have access to ultrasound scanning of the renal tract out of hours or at the weekend.

Only 177/297 (60%) of all hospitals were able to provide a nephrostomy service out of hours during the week. This figure was similar for the weekend (170/291: 58%)

Only a small proportion of hospitals providing RRT in level 2/3 units had input from a nephrologist.

Recommendations

All acute admitting hospitals should have access to either onsite nephrologists or a dedicated nephrology service within reasonable distance of the admitting hospital. (Clinical Directors and Medical Directors)

All acute admitting hospitals should have access to a renal ultrasound scanning service 24 hours a day including the weekends and the ability to provide emergency relief of renal obstruction. (Clinical Directors and Medical Directors)

All level 3 units should have the ability to deliver renal replacement therapy; and where appropriate these patients should receive clinical input from a nephrologist. (Clinical Directors and Medical Directors)

Conclusion

In this study NCEPOD has uncovered systematic failings in the management of AKI. These largely relate to the failure of clinicians to recognise and manage the condition appropriately. It is important to remember that all the patients in this study died with a primary diagnosis of acute kidney injury thus it is reasonable to surmise that, in at least some cases, the outcome for the patient may have been different if the condition had been recognised and managed better.

There was also a failure to recognise the complications of AKI; the condition was often recognised late thus complications were more likely to be present. This did not stop those complications being missed or badly managed. In other words AKI was overlooked, poorly assessed and when eventually recognised mismanaged in this group of patients.

The fact is that the very basics of medical care were being omitted. Regular checks on biochemistry, administration of IV fluids and fluid balance measurements are not central to basic management plans. This inevitably makes the recommendations made appear trite. However, NCEPOD firmly believes that unless attention is paid to the basics, the prevalence and outcome of this condition in hospital patients will not improve. Whilst there are undoubtedly some organisational issues to be addressed there are many more clinical issues.

Many of these issues are around the recognition of the acutely ill patient; an area that NCEPOD has visited in previous reports[3,8]. Thus the clinical failures in AKI management are really a microcosm of a more global failure of the sick patient by hospital staff. Perhaps then, it is more pertinent to argue that unless the recognition and management of the acutely ill patient is improved there is little chance of correcting deficiencies around AKI. To this end we hope that this report informs the debate not only around acute kidney injury but also acute patient care in its totality.

References

1. Naikar SS, Liu KD, Chertow GM. The incidence and prognostic significance of acute kidney injury. Cherow 2007. Curr Opin Nep Nephrol Hypertens; 16:227-236.

2. Hoste EA, Clermont G, Kersten A, et al. RIFLE criteria for acute kidney injury are associated with hospital mortality in critically ill patients: a cohort analysis. 2006. Crit Care. 10(3):R73.

3. Emergency Admissions: A journey in the right direction? 2007. National Confidential Enquiry into Patient Outcome and Death. London. http://www.ncepod.org.uk/reports.htm

4. Dwinnell BG and Anderson RJ. Diagnostic Evaluation of the Patient with Acute Renal Failure, Chapter 12. http://www.kidneyatlas.org/book1/adk1_12.pdf

5. Bion JF and Heffner JE. Challenges in the care of the acutely ill. 2004. Lancet 363:970-977.

6. Franklin C and Mathew J. Developing strategies to prevent in-hospital cardiac arrest: analyzing responses of physicians and nurses in the hours before the event. 1994. Crit Care Med 22:244-247.

7. McQuillan P, Pilkington S, Allan A, et al. Confidential inquiry into quality of care before admission to intensive care. 1998. BMJ 316:1853-1858.

8. An Acute Problem. 2005. National Confidential Enquiry into Patient Outcome and Death. http://www.ncepod.org.uk/2005report/

9. Stevens PE, Tamimi NA, Al Hasani MK, et al. Non-specialist management of acute renal failure. 2001. QJM 94: 533–540.

10. Vijayan A and Miller SB. Acute renal failure: prevention and nondialytic therapy. 1998. Semin Nephrol 18:523-532.

11. Davidman M, Olson P, Kohen J, et al. Iatrogenic renal disease. 1991. Arch Intern Med 151:1809-1812.

12. The Renal Association. 2008. Clinical Practice Guideline 10.3-AKI: Nutritional Support.

13. Uchino, S, Doig, GS, Bellomo, R, et al. Diuretics and mortality in acute renal failure. 2004. Crit Care Med 32:1669-1677.

14. Kellum, JA and Decker, JM Use of dopamine in acute renal failure: a meta-analysis. 2001. Crit Care Med 29:1526-1531.

15. Marik, PE. Low-dose dopamine: a systematic review. 2002. Intensive Care Med. 28:877-883.

16. Friedrich, JO, Adhikari, N, Herridge, MS, et al. Meta-analysis: low-dose dopamine increases urine output but does not prevent renal dysfunction or death. 2005. Ann Intern Med 142:510-524.

17. Bellomo, R, Chapman, M, Finfer, S, et al. Low-dose dopamine in patients with early renal dysfunction: a placebo-controlled randomised trial. 2000. Australian and New Zealand Intensive Care Society (ANZICS) Clinical Trials Group. Lancet 356:2139-2143.

18. Khan IH, Catto GR, Edward N, et al. Acute renal failure: factors influencing nephrology referral and outcome. 1997. QJM. 90(12):781-5.

19. The National Service Framework for Renal Services-Part Two: Chronic Kidney Disease, Acute Renal Failure and End of Life Care. 2005. Department of Health.

20. Feest TG, Mistry CD, Grimes DS, et al. Incidence of advanced chronic kidney disease and the need for end stage renal replacement therapy. 1990. BMJ 301:897–900.

21. Khan IH, Catto GRD, Edward N, et al. Chronic kidney disease: factors influencing nephrology referral. 1994. QJ M 87:559–64.

22. Parry R G, Crowe A, Stevens J M, et al. Referral of elderly patients with severe renal failure: questionnaire survey of physicians. 1996. BMJ 313:466.

23. Pannu N, Klarenbach S, Wiebe N, et al. Renal replacement therapy in patients with acute renal failure: a systematic review. 2008. JAMA. 299(7):793-805.

24. Rabindranath K, Adams J, Macleod AM, et al. Intermittent versus continuous renal replacement therapy for acute renal failure in adults. 2007. Cochrane Database Syst Rev. 18;(3):CD003773.

25. Withholding and Withdrawing Life-prolonging Treatments: Good Practice in Decision-making. 2002. General Medical Council.

26. http://www.dh.gov.uk/en/SocialCare/Deliveringadult socialcare/MentalCapacity/IMCA/index.htm).

27. McQuillan P, Pilkington S, Allan A et al. Confidential inquiry into quality of care before admission to intensive care. 1998. BMJ 316:1853-1858.

28. McGloin H, Adam SK and Singer M. Unexpected deaths and referrals to intensive care of patients on general wards. Are some cases potentially avoidable? 1999. J R Coll Physicians Lond 33(3):255-259.

29. Seward E, Greig E, Preston S, et al. A confidential study of deaths after emergency medical admission: issues relating to quality of care. 2003. Clin Med 3(5):425-434.

30. Franklin C, Mathew J. Developing strategies to prevent in-hospital cardiac arrest: analyzing responses of physicians and nurses in the hours before the event. 1994. Crit Care Med 22(2):244-247.

31. Schein RM, Hazday N, Pena M, et al. Clinical antecedents to in-hospital cardiopulmonary arrest. 1990. Chest 98(6):1388-1392.

Appendices

Appendix 1 – Glossary

AKI	Acute kidney injury
CKD	Chronic kidney disease
CPAP	Continuous positive airway pressure
CT	Computed tomography
CVP	Central venous pressure
DNAR	Do not attempt resuscitation
GFR	Glomerular filtration rate
GP	General Practitioner
ICD10	International classification of disease
LFT	Liver function tests
MEWS	Modified early warning score
NCEPOD	National Confidential Enquiry into Patient Outcome and Death
NICE	National Institute for Health and Clinical Excellence
NSAIDs	Non-steroidal, anti-inflammatory drugs
RCT	Randomised controlled trial
RIFLE	Risk, Injury, Failure, Loss, End-stage kidney disease
RRT	Renal replacement therapy
ST	Specialist Trainee
SpR	Specialist Registrar
TPR	Temperature, pulse, respiratory rate
U & E	Urea and electrolytes

Appendix 2 – RIFLE Classification

Risk, Injury, Failure, Loss, and End-stage kidney disease (RIFLE) classification

Class	GFR criteria	UO criteria
Risk	Serum creatinine x 1.5	<0.5 ml/kg/h x 6 h
Injury	Serum creatinine x 2	<0.5 ml/kg/h x 12 h
Failure	Serum creatinine x 3 or serum creatinine ≥ 4 mg/dl with an acute rise >0.5 mg/dl	<0.3 ml/kg/h x 24 h or anuria x 12 h
Loss	Persistent acute renal failure = complete loss of kidney function >4 weeks	
End-stage kidney disease	End-stage kidney disease >3 months	

For conversion of creatinine expressed in conventional units to ST units, multiply by 88.4. Patients are categorized on serum creatinine or urinary output (UO), or both, and the criteria that led to the worst classification are used. Glomerular filtration rate (GFR) criteria are calculated as an increase of serum creatinine above the baseline serum creatinine level. When the baseline serum creatinine is unknown and there is no past history of chronic kidney disease, serum creatinine is calculated using the Modification of Diet in Renal Disease formula for assessment of kidney function, assuming a glomerular filtration rate of 75 ml/minute/1.73 m^2. Acute kidney injury should be considered when kidney dysfunction is abrupt (within 1 to 7 days) and sustained (more than 24 hours).

Lopes et al. Critical Care 2006 11:401 doi:10.1186/cc5121

Appendix 3 – Classification of renal failure

Mode of presentation	Inclusion criteria
Acute renal failure	Presented unexpectedly with normal sized kidneys, or presented after known renal insult, previous renal function normal, or presented after known renal insult, previous function unknown but normal size kidneys
Acute-on-chronic	Presented either unexpectedly or after a known renal insult and known to have had previous serum creatinine > 150 mmol/l, or shown ultrasound to have at least one small kidney (< 8 cm)
Chronic renal failure	Known to have had chronic renal failure followed by a physician, no obvious renal insult precipitating requirement for dialysis

CKD Stage	Estimated GFR	Urine output criteria
1	90+	Normal kidney function but urine findings or structural abnormalities or genetic trait point to kidney disease
2	60-89	Mildly reduced kidney function and other findings (as stage 1) point to kidney disease
3	30-59	Moderatly reduced kidney function
4	15-29	Severley reduced kidney function
5	<15	Very severe or endstage kidney failure (sometimes called established renal failure)

AKI Stage	Serum creatinine criteria	Urine output criteria
1	Increase in serum creatinine of more than 0.3 mg/dl ($\geq$ 26.4 µmol/l or increase to more than or equal to 150% to 200% (1.5- to 2-fold) from baseline	Less than 0.5 ml/kg per hour for more than 6 hours
2	Increase in serum creatinine to more than 200% to 300% (> 2- to 3-fold) from baseline	Less than 0.5 ml/kg per hour for more than 12 hours
3	Incease in serum creatinine to more than 300% (> 3-fold) from baseline (or serum creatinine of more than or equal to 4.0 mg/dl (> 354 µmol/l) with an acute increase of at least 0.5 mg/dl (44 µmol/l)	Less than 0.3 ml/kg per hour for 24 hours or anuria for 12 hours

Appendix 4

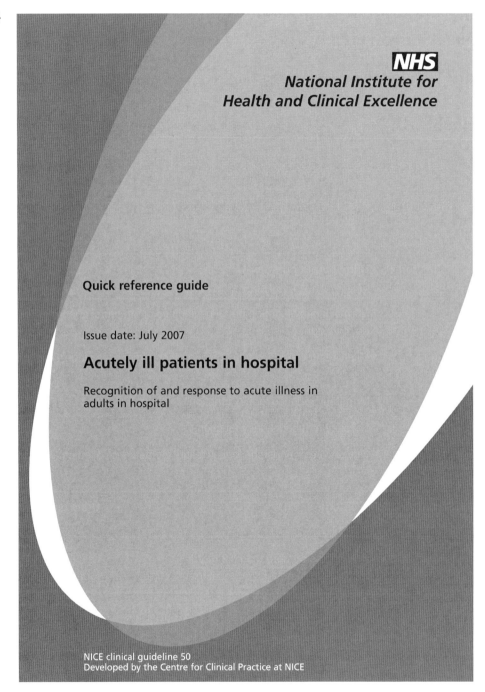

Acutely ill patients in hospital

Contents

Introduction

Any patient in hospital may become acutely ill. However, the recognition of acute illness is often delayed and its subsequent management may be inappropriate. This may result in late referral and avoidable admissions to critical care, and may lead to unnecessary patient deaths, particularly when the initial standard of care is suboptimal.

The NICE clinical guideline makes evidence-based recommendations on the recognition and management of acute illness in acute hospitals. More information, including the evidence from which the recommendations were derived, is available from www.nice.org.uk/CG050

Patient-centred care

Treatment and care should take into account patients' individual needs and preferences. Good communication is essential, supported by evidence-based information, to allow patients to reach informed decisions about their care. If the patient agrees, carers and relatives should have the opportunity to be involved in decisions about treatment and care.

National Institute for
Health and Clinical Excellence
MidCity Place
71 High Holborn
London
WC1V 6NA

www.nice.org.uk

ISBN 1-84629-440-1

This guidance is written in the following context
This guidance represents the view of the Institute, which was arrived at after careful consideration of the evidence available. Healthcare professionals are expected to take it fully into account when exercising their clinical judgement. The guidance does not, however, override the individual responsibility of healthcare professionals to make decisions appropriate to the circumstances of the individual patient, in consultation with the patient and/or guardian or carer.

Key priorities for implementation

- Adult patients in acute hospital settings, including patients in the emergency department for whom a clinical decision to admit has been made, should have:
  - physiological observations recorded at the time of their admission or initial assessment
  - a clear written monitoring plan that specifies which physiological observations should be recorded and how often. The plan should take account of the:
    - patient's diagnosis
    - presence of comorbidities
    - agreed treatment plan.

  Physiological observations should be recorded and acted upon by staff who have been trained to undertake these procedures and understand their clinical relevance.

- Physiological track and trigger systems should be used to monitor all adult patients in acute hospital settings.
  - Physiological observations should be monitored at least every 12 hours, unless a decision has been made at a senior level to increase or decrease this frequency for an individual patient.
  - The frequency of monitoring should increase if abnormal physiology is detected, as outlined in the recommendation on graded response strategy.

- Staff caring for patients in acute hospital settings should have competencies in monitoring, measurement, interpretation and prompt response to the acutely ill patient appropriate to the level of care they are providing. Education and training should be provided to ensure staff have these competencies, and they should be assessed to ensure they can demonstrate them.

- A graded response strategy for patients identified as being at risk of clinical deterioration should be agreed and delivered locally. It should consist of the following three levels.
  - Low-score group:
    - Increased frequency of observations and the nurse in charge alerted.
  - Medium-score group:
    - Urgent call to team with primary medical responsibility for the patient.
    - Simultaneous call to personnel with core competencies for acute illness. These competencies can be delivered by a variety of models at a local level, such as a critical care outreach team, a hospital-at-night team or a specialist trainee in an acute medical or surgical specialty.
  - High-score group:
    - Emergency call to team with critical care competencies and diagnostic skills. The team should include a medical practitioner skilled in the assessment of the critically ill patient, who possesses advanced airway management and resuscitation skills. There should be an immediate response.

- If the team caring for the patient considers that admission to a critical care area is clinically indicated, then the decision to admit should involve both the consultant caring for the patient on the ward and the consultant in critical care.

Continued on page 6

Acutely ill patients in hospital

Recognition of and response to acute illness in adults in hospital

Recognition of and response to acute illness in adults in hospital

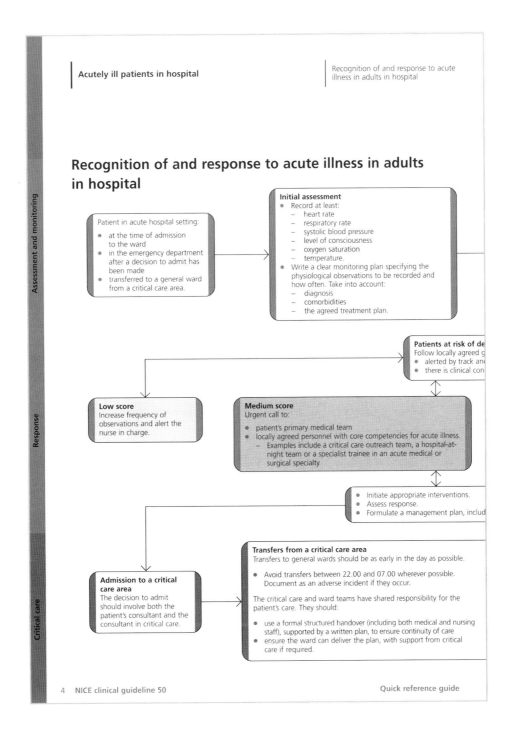

Assessment and monitoring

Patient in acute hospital setting:

- at the time of admission to the ward
- in the emergency department after a decision to admit has been made
- transferred to a general ward from a critical care area.

Initial assessment
- Record at least:
  - heart rate
  - respiratory rate
  - systolic blood pressure
  - level of consciousness
  - oxygen saturation
  - temperature.
- Write a clear monitoring plan specifying the physiological observations to be recorded and how often. Take into account:
  - diagnosis
  - comorbidities
  - the agreed treatment plan.

Patients at risk of de
Follow locally agreed g
- alerted by track an
- there is clinical con

Response

Low score
Increase frequency of observations and alert the nurse in charge.

Medium score
Urgent call to:

- patient's primary medical team
- locally agreed personnel with core competencies for acute illness.
  - Examples include a critical care outreach team, a hospital-at-night team or a specialist trainee in an acute medical or surgical specialty.

- Initiate appropriate interventions.
- Assess response.
- Formulate a management plan, includ

Critical care

Admission to a critical care area
The decision to admit should involve both the patient's consultant and the consultant in critical care.

Transfers from a critical care area
Transfers to general wards should be as early in the day as possible.

- Avoid transfers between 22.00 and 07.00 wherever possible. Document as an adverse incident if they occur.

The critical care and ward teams have shared responsibility for the patient's care. They should:

- use a formal structured handover (including both medical and nursing staff), supported by a written plan, to ensure continuity of care
- ensure the ward can deliver the plan, with support from critical care if required.

Acutely ill patients in hospital

Recognition of and response to acute illness in adults in hospital

Routine monitoring
Use physiological track and trigger systems to monitor patients.

- Monitor physiological observations at least every 12 hours, unless decided at a senior level to increase or decrease the frequency for an individual patient.
- Use multiple-parameter or aggregate weighted scoring systems, which allow a graded response. The systems should:
  – define the parameters to be measured and the frequency of observations
  – state the parameters, cut-off points or scores that should trigger a response
  – monitor:
    ◆ heart rate
    ◆ respiratory rate

    ◆ systolic blood pressure
    ◆ level of consciousness
    ◆ oxygen saturation
    ◆ temperature.

- Set thresholds locally, and review regularly to optimise sensitivity and specificity.

Consider monitoring:

- biochemistry (for example, lactate, blood glucose, base deficit, arterial pH)
- hourly urine output
- pain.

…erioration
…aded response strategy if:
…trigger score
…ern.

Clinical emergency (excluding cardiac arrests).

High score
Emergency call to team with critical care competencies and diagnostic skills. The team should:

- include a medical practitioner skilled in assessing critically ill patients and with advanced airway management and resuscitation skills
- provide an immediate response.

Staff competencies
Physiological observations should be recorded and acted upon by staff specifically trained to undertake them and understand their clinical relevance.

Staff should have competencies, appropriate to the level of care they provide, in:

- monitoring
- measurement
- interpretation
- prompt response.

These should be assessed, and education and training provided.

Ward staff working with patients transferred from critical care areas should be educated to recognise and understand their physical, psychological and emotional needs.

…g location and level of care.

The handover of care should include:

- a summary of the critical care stay including diagnosis and treatment
- a monitoring and investigation plan
- a plan for ongoing treatment including drugs and therapies, nutrition plan, infection status and any agreed limitations of treatment
- physical and rehabilitation needs
- psychological and emotional needs
- specific communication or language needs.

Staff should offer patients information about their condition and encourage them to participate in decisions that relate to their recovery.

NICE clinical guideline 50

Quick reference guide   5

Assessment and monitoring

Response

Critical care

Key priorities for implementation *continued*

- After the decision to transfer a patient from a critical care area to the general ward has been made, he or she should be transferred as early as possible during the day. Transfer from critical care areas to the general ward between 22.00 and 07.00 should be avoided whenever possible, and should be documented as an adverse incident if it occurs.

- The critical care area transferring team and the receiving ward team should take shared responsibility for the care of the patient being transferred. They should jointly ensure:
  - there is continuity of care through a formal structured handover of care from critical care area staff to ward staff (including both medical and nursing staff), supported by a written plan
  - that the receiving ward, with support from critical care if required, can deliver the agreed plan.

  The formal structured handover of care should include:
  - a summary of critical care stay, including diagnosis and treatment
  - a monitoring and investigation plan
  - a plan for ongoing treatment, including drugs and therapies, nutrition plan, infection status and any agreed limitations of treatment
  - physical and rehabilitation needs
  - psychological and emotional needs
  - specific communication or language needs.

Implementation

NICE has developed tools to help organisations implement this guidance (listed below). These are available on our website (www.nice.org.uk/CG050).

● Slides highlighting key messages for local discussion.

● Implementation advice on how to put the guidance into practice and national initiatives which support this locally.

● Costing tools:
 – costing report to estimate the national savings and costs associated with implementation
 – costing template to estimate the local costs and savings involved.

● Audit criteria to monitor local practice.

Further information

Ordering information

You can download the following documents from www.nice.org.uk/CG050

● A quick reference guide (this document) – a summary of the recommendations for healthcare professionals.

● 'Understanding NICE guidance' – information for patients and carers.

● The full guideline – all the recommendations, details of how they were developed, and summaries of the evidence they were based on.

For printed copies of the quick reference guide or 'Understanding NICE guidance', phone the NHS Response Line on 0870 1555 455 and quote:

● N1287 (quick reference guide)

● N1288 ('Understanding NICE guidance').

Related NICE guidance

For information about NICE guidance that has been issued or is in development, see the website (www.nice.org.uk).

● Nutrition support in adults: oral nutrition support, enteral tube feeding and parenteral nutrition. NICE clinical guideline 32 (2006). Available from: www.nice.org.uk/CG032

Updating the guideline

This guideline will be updated as needed, and information about the progress of any update will be posted on the NICE website (www.nice.org/CG050).

About this booklet

This is a quick reference guide that summarises the recommendations NICE has made to the NHS in Acutely ill patients in hospital: recognition of and response to acute illness in adults in hospital (NICE clinical guideline 50).

Who should read this booklet?

This quick reference guide is for nurses, doctors, therapists and other staff who care for acutely ill patients. It contains what you need to know to put the guideline's recommendations into practice.

Who wrote the guideline?

The guideline was developed by the Centre for Clinical Practice at NICE following the short clinical guideline process. The Centre worked with an independent group of healthcare professionals (including consultants from relevant specialties and nurses), patients and carers, and technical staff, who reviewed the evidence and drafted the recommendations. The recommendations were finalised after public consultation.

For more information on how NICE clinical guidelines are developed, go to www.nice.org.uk

Where can I get more information about the guideline on acutely ill patients in hospital?

The NICE website has the recommendations in full with summaries of the evidence they are based on, a summary of the guideline for patients and carers, and tools to support implementation (see inside back cover for more details).

**National Institute for
Health and Clinical Excellence**

MidCity Place
71 High Holborn
London
WC1V 6NA

www.nice.org.uk

N1287 1P 50k Jul 07

ISBN 1-84629-440-1

Appendix 5 – Modified Early Warning Score (MEWS)

MEWS Score	3	2	1	0	1	2	3
Pulse		≤ 40	41-50	51-100	101-110	111-130	≥ 131
Respiratory		≤ 8		9-14	15-20	21-29	≥ 30
Temperature		≤ 35	35.1-36	36.1-38	38.1-38.5	≥ 38.6	
AVPU	Completely unresponsive	Pain	Voice	Alert	New agilation or confusion		
Glasgow Coma Score				15	14	9-13	≤ 8
Urine Output	< 10ml/h	< 20ml/h					
Syatolic BP	< 70	71-80	81-100	101-199		> 200	

AVPU is a simple assement where: A = Alert
V = Responds to verbal commands only
P = Responds to Pain
U = Completely unresponsive

The Glasgow Coma Scale (GCS) is an alternative to AVPU but should only be used at the discretion of the Medical Team.

- A MEWS must be calculated where a patient scores 2 or more in ANY observation category
- At the initial stage MEWS observations should be calculated and recorded at $1/2$ hourly intervals (this may be changed to less frequent intervals after formal medical review of the patient)
- A MEWS of 4 or more and/or a MEWS increase of 2 or more MUST trigger an urgent referral of medical review

- During daytime hours nursing staff should initiate a MEWS Call to the relevant speciality team (e.g. Surgical or Medical Registrar). Out of hours this should be to the Clinical Site Manager
- If there is no response to the initial MEWS call within 10 minutes, nursing staff should initiate a fast-bleep to the Speciality Team (or Clinical Site Manager out of hours) via Switchboard
- A member of medical staff MUST attend and assess the patient within 30 minutes.

APPENDICES

Appendix 6 – Corporate Structure

The National Confidential Enquiry into Patient Outcome and Death (NCEPOD) is an independent body to which a corporate commitment has been made by the Medical and Surgical Colleges, Associations and Faculties related to its area of activity. Each of these bodies nominates members on to NCEPOD's Steering Group.

Steering Group as at 11th June 2009

Dr D Whitaker	Association of Anaesthetists of Great Britain and Ireland
Mr T Bates	Association of Surgeons of Great Britain & Ireland
Mr J Wardrope	College of Emergency Medicine
Dr S Bridgman	Faculty of Public Health Medicine of the United Kingdom
Dr P Cartwright	Royal College of Anaesthetists
Dr P Nightingale	Royal College of Anaesthetists
Dr B Ellis	Royal College of General Practitioners
Ms M McElligott	Royal College of Nursing
Prof D Luesley	Royal College of Obstetricians and Gynaecologists
Mrs M Wishart	Royal College of Ophthalmologists
Dr I Doughty	Royal College of Paediatrics and Child Health
Dr R Dowdle	Royal College of Physicians
Professor T Hendra	Royal College of Physicians
Dr M Armitage	Royal College of Physicians
Dr M Clements	Royal College of Physicians
Dr S McPherson	Royal College of Radiologists
Mr B Rees	Royal College of Surgeons of England
Mr M Parker	Royal College of Surgeons of England
Mr D Mitchell	Faculty of Dental Surgery, Royal College of Surgeons of England
Vacancy	Royal College of Pathologists
Ms S Panizzo	Patient Representative
Mrs M Wang	Patient Representative

Observers

Mrs C Miles	Institute of Healthcare Management
Dr R Palmer	Coroners' Society of England and Wales
Mrs H Burton	Scottish Audit of Surgical Mortality
Dr K Cleary	National Patient Safety Agency
Ms R Brown	National Patient Safety Agency
Professor P Littlejohns	National Institute for Health and Clinical Excellence

NCEPOD is a company, limited by guarantee and a registered charity, managed by Trustees.

Trustees

Professor T Treasure (Chairman)
Professor G T Layer (Honorary Treasurer)
Professor M Britton
Professor J H Shepherd
Mr M A M S Leigh
Dr D Justins

Dr M Mason (Company Secretary)

Clinical Co-ordinators

The Steering Group appoint a Lead Clinical Co-ordinator for a defined tenure. In addition there are seven Clinical Co-ordinators who work on each study. All Co-ordinators are engaged in active clinical/academic practice (in the NHS) during their term of office.

Lead Clinical Co-ordinator	Mr I C Martin (Surgery)
Clinical Co-ordinators	Dr D G Mason (Anaesthesia)
	Dr K Wilkinson (Anaesthesia)
	Dr A Goodwin (Anaesthesia)
	Dr J A D Stewart (Medicine)
	Professor S B Lucas (Pathology)
	Dr G Findlay (Intensive Care)
	Mr M Gough (Surgery)

Appendix 7 – Participation

Organisation	Death data	Clinical Q sent	Clinical Q returned	Casenotes returned	Organis- ational Q returned
Abertawe Bro Morgannwg University NHS Trust	Yes	17	3	2	Yes
Aintree Hospitals NHS Foundation Trust	Yes	16	10	10	Yes
Airedale NHS Trust	Yes	2	2	2	Yes
Ashford & St Peter's Hospital NHS Trust	Yes	2	2	2	Yes
Aspen Healthcare	Yes	0	0	0	Yes
Barking, Havering and Redbridge Hospitals NHS Trust	Yes	9	8	8	Yes
Barnet and Chase Farm Hospitals NHS Trust	Yes	5	1	1	Yes
Barnsley Hospital NHS Foundation Trust	Yes	6	2	1	Yes
Barts and The London NHS Trust	Yes	6	2	1	Yes
Basildon & Thurrock University Hospitals NHS FoundationTrust	Yes	6	6	5	Yes
Basingstoke & North Hampshire Hospitals NHS Foundation Trust	Yes	3	3	2	No
Bedford Hospital NHS Trust	Yes	10	3	3	Yes
Belfast Health and Social Care Trust	Yes	13	9	6	Yes
Birmingham Women's Healthcare NHS Trust	No	0	0	0	Yes
Blackpool, Fylde and Wyre Hospitals NHS Foundation Trust	Yes	8	5	4	Yes
BMI Healthcare	Yes	1	1	1	Yes
Bolton Hospitals NHS Trust	Yes	8	7	5	Yes
Bradford Teaching Hospitals NHS Foundation Trust	Yes	7	4	3	Yes
Brighton and Sussex University Hospitals NHS Trust	Yes	12	11	12	Yes
Bromley Hospitals NHS Trust	Yes	3	2	2	Yes
Buckinghamshire Hospitals NHS Trust	Yes	1	1	1	Yes
Burton Hospitals NHS Foundation Trust	Yes	5	4	4	Yes
Calderdale & Huddersfield NHS Foundation Trust	No	0	0	0	Yes
Cambridge University Hospitals NHS Foundation Trust	Yes	0	0	0	Yes
Cardiff and Vale NHS Trust	No	0	0	0	Yes
Care UK	No	0	0	0	Yes
Central Manchester University Hospitals NHS Foundation Trust	Yes	2	2	0	Yes
Chelsea & Westminster Healthcare NHS Trust	Yes	3	3	3	Yes
Chesterfield Royal Hospital NHS Foundation Trust	Yes	2	2	2	Yes
City Hospitals Sunderland NHS Foundation Trust	Yes	9	9	9	Yes
Clatterbridge Centre for Oncology NHS Trust	Yes	0	0	0	Yes
Colchester Hospital University NHS Foundation Trust	Yes	5	5	5	Yes
Countess of Chester Hospital NHS Foundation Trust	Yes	14	9	6	Yes

Participation continued

Organisation	Death data	Clinical Q sent	Clinical Q returned	Casenotes returned	Organis- ational Q returned
County Durham and Darlington NHS Foundation Trust	Yes	14	11	9	Yes
Cwm Taf NHS Trust	Yes	7	4	2	No
Dartford & Gravesham NHS Trust	Yes	8	5	4	Yes
Derby Hospitals NHS Foundation Trust	Yes	5	5	2	No
Doncaster and Bassetlaw Hospitals NHS Foundation Trust	Yes	11	8	4	Yes
Dorset County Hospital NHS Foundation Trust	Yes	4	4	4	Yes
Dudley Group of Hospitals NHS Trust	Yes	14	2	2	No
Ealing Hospital NHS Trust	Yes	3	3	2	Yes
East & North Hertfordshire NHS Trust	Yes	9	6	6	No
East Cheshire NHS Trust	Yes	6	5	1	No
East Kent Hospitals NHS Trust	Yes	18	9	8	Yes
East Lancashire Hospitals NHS Trust	Yes	4	2	1	Yes
East Sussex Hospitals NHS Trust	Yes	16	14	13	Yes
Epsom and St Helier University Hospitals NHS Trust	Yes	18	9	4	Yes
Frimley Park Hospitals NHS Trust	Yes	9	5	6	Yes
Gateshead Health NHS Foundation Trust	Yes	8	6	7	No
George Eliot Hospital NHS Trust	Yes	7	2	0	No
Gloucestershire Hospitals NHS Foundation Trust	Yes	6	3	1	Yes
Great Western Hospitals NHS Foundation Trust	Yes	4	4	4	Yes
Guy's & St Thomas' NHS Foundation Trust	Yes	8	3	0	Yes
Gwent Healthcare NHS Trust	No	0	0	0	No
Harrogate and District NHS Foundation Trust	Yes	1	1	1	Yes
HCA International	Yes	0	0	0	Yes
Health & Social Services, States of Guernsey	Yes	0	0	0	Yes
Heart of England NHS Foundation Trust	Yes	21	11	9	Yes
Heatherwood & Wexham Park Hospitals NHS Foundation Trust	Yes	5	4	4	Yes
Hereford Hospitals NHS Trust	Yes	1	1	1	Yes
Hillingdon Hospital NHS Trust	Yes	2	2	2	Yes
Hinchingbrooke Health Care NHS Trust	No	0	0	0	Yes
Homerton University Hospital NHS Foundation Trust	Yes	2	2	2	Yes
Hospital of St John and St Elizabeth	Yes	0	0	0	Yes
Hull and East Yorkshire Hospitals NHS Trust	Yes	0	0	0	No
Hywel Dda NHS Trust	Yes	5	4	3	Yes
Imperial College Healthcare NHS Trust	Yes	11	6	4	Yes
Ipswich Hospital NHS Trust	Yes	7	3	3	Yes

Participation continued

Organisation	Death data	Clinical Q sent	Clinical Q returned	Casenotes returned	Organis- ational Q returned
Isle of Man Department of Health & Social Security	Yes	2	2	2	Yes
Isle of Wight Healthcare NHS Trust	Yes	2	0	1	Yes
James Paget Healthcare NHS Trust	Yes	8	5	5	Yes
Kettering General Hospital NHS Trust	Yes	5	5	5	Yes
King Edward VII's Hospital Sister Agnes	Yes	0	0	0	Yes
King's College Hospital NHS Trust	Yes	5	2	3	Yes
Kingston Hospital NHS Trust	Yes	8	6	5	Yes
Lancashire Teaching Hospitals NHS Foundation Trust	Yes	13	9	5	Yes
Leeds Teaching Hospitals NHS Trust (The)	Yes	16	7	5	Yes
Lewisham Hospital NHS Trust	Yes	3	3	2	Yes
Liverpool Heart and Chest Hospital NHS Trust	Yes	0	0	0	Yes
Liverpool Women's NHS Foundation Trust	No	0	0	0	Yes
London Clinic	No	0	0	0	Yes
Luton and Dunstable Hospital NHS Foundation Trust	Yes	14	4	3	Yes
Maidstone and Tunbridge Wells NHS Trust	Yes	8	2	1	No
Mayday Health Care NHS Trust	Yes	10	7	7	Yes
Medway NHS Trust	Yes	4	1	1	Yes
Mid Cheshire Hospitals NHS Trust	Yes	4	2	2	Yes
Mid Staffordshire General Hospitals NHS Trust	Yes	11	10	8	Yes
Mid Yorkshire Hospitals NHS Trust	Yes	20	14	20	Yes
Mid-Essex Hospital Services NHS Trust	Yes	7	5	3	Yes
Milton Keynes Hospital NHS Foundation Trust	Yes	3	3	2	Yes
Netcare Healthcare UK Ltd	No	0	0	0	Yes
Newcastle upon Tyne Hospitals NHS Foundation Trust	Yes	11	11	10	Yes
Newham University Hospital NHS Trust	Yes	2	1	1	No
Norfolk & Norwich University Hospital NHS Trust	Yes	9	7	6	Yes
North Bristol NHS Trust	Yes	13	11	12	Yes
North Cumbria Acute Hospitals NHS Trust	Yes	8	7	6	Yes
North Middlesex University Hospital NHS Trust	Yes	3	3	2	No
North Tees and Hartlepool NHS Foundation Trust	Yes	2	1	1	Yes
North Wales NHS Trust	Yes	6	4	4	Yes
North West London Hospitals NHS Trust	Yes	1	1	1	Yes
North West Wales NHS Trust	Yes	0	0	0	No
Northampton General Hospital NHS Trust	Yes	2	2	2	Yes
Northern Devon Healthcare NHS Trust	Yes	2	0	0	Yes
Northern Health & Social CareTrust	No	0	0	0	Yes
Northern Lincolnshire & Goole Hospitals Trust	Yes	6	4	3	Yes

Participation continued

Organisation	Death data	Clinical Q sent	Clinical Q returned	Casenotes returned	Organis-ational Q returned
Northumbria Healthcare NHS Trust	Yes	7	4	3	Yes
Nottingham University Hospitals NHS Trust	Yes	16	10	9	Yes
Nuffield Health	Yes	0	0	0	Yes
Oxford Radcliffe Hospital NHS Trust	Yes	3	3	3	Yes
Papworth Hospital NHS Foundation Trust	No	0	0	0	Yes
Pennine Acute Hospitals NHS Trust (The)	Yes	27	13	27	Yes
Peterborough & Stamford Hospitals NHS Foundation Trust	Yes	8	7	7	Yes
Plymouth Hospitals NHS Trust	Yes	9	8	6	Yes
Poole Hospital NHS Trust	Yes	9	7	5	Yes
Portsmouth Hospitals NHS Trust	Yes	0	0	0	Yes
Princess Alexandra Hospital NHS Trust	Yes	7	4	2	No
Princess Mary's Hospital	No	0	0	0	No
Queen Elizabeth Hospital NHS Trust	Yes	1	0	0	Yes
Queen Mary's Sidcup NHS Trust	Yes	6	5	4	Yes
Queen Victoria Hospital NHS Foundation Trust	Yes	0	0	0	Yes
Ramsay Health Care UK	Yes	0	0	0	Yes
Robert Jones and Agnes Hunt Orthopaedic & District Hospital	Yes	0	0	0	No
Royal Berkshire NHS Foundation Trust	Yes	3	3	3	Yes
Royal Bournemouth and Christchurch Hospitals NHS Trust	Yes	5	5	4	Yes
Royal Brompton and Harefield NHS Trust	Yes	0	0	0	No
Royal Cornwall Hospitals NHS Trust	Yes	8	7	8	Yes
Royal Devon and Exeter NHS Foundation Trust	Yes	10	10	10	Yes
Royal Free Hampstead NHS Trust	Yes	2	2	2	Yes
Royal Liverpool & Broadgreen University Hospitals NHS Trust	Yes	10	7	7	Yes
Royal Marsden NHS Foundation Trust (The)	Yes	0	0	0	Yes
Royal Orthopaedic Hospital NHS Foundation Trust	Yes	0	0	0	Yes
Royal Surrey County Hospital NHS Trust	Yes	1	1	1	Yes
Royal United Hospital Bath NHS Trust	Yes	3	1	1	No
Royal West Sussex NHS Trust	Yes	5	1	1	Yes
Royal Wolverhampton Hospitals NHS Trust (The)	Yes	11	6	6	No
Salford Royal Hospitals NHS Foundation Trust	Yes	3	2	3	Yes
Salisbury Foundation NHS Trust	Yes	0	0	0	Yes
Sandwell and West Birmingham Hospitals NHS Trust	Yes	13	13	12	Yes

Participation continued

Organisation	Death data	Clinical Q sent	Clinical Q returned	Casenotes returned	Organis- ational Q returned
Scarborough and North East Yorkshire Health Care NHS Trust	No	0	0	0	Yes
Sheffield Teaching Hospitals NHS Foundation Trust	Yes	23	18	19	Yes
Sherwood Forest Hospitals NHS Trust	Yes	6	6	6	Yes
Shrewsbury and Telford Hospitals NHS Trust	Yes	6	6	6	Yes
South Devon Healthcare NHS Foundation Trust	Yes	5	5	4	Yes
South Downs Health NHS Trust	No	0	0	0	No
South Eastern Health & Social Care Trust	Yes	0	0	0	Yes
South Tees Hospitals NHS Trust	Yes	8	8	8	Yes
South Tyneside NHS Foundation Trust	Yes	6	5	3	Yes
South Warwickshire General Hospitals NHS Trust	Yes	2	2	2	Yes
Southampton University Hospitals NHS Trust	Yes	3	3	2	Yes
Southend University Hospital NHS Foundation Trust	Yes	4	2	0	No
Southern Health & Social Care Trust	Yes	3	2	1	Yes
Southport and Ormskirk Hospitals NHS Trust	Yes	2	2	1	Yes
Spire Healthcare	Yes	0	0	0	Yes
St Anthony's Hospital	Yes	0	0	0	No
St George's Healthcare NHS Trust	Yes	1	1	1	Yes
St Helens and Knowsley Teaching Hospitals NHS Trust	Yes	10	10	9	Yes
States of Jersey Health & Social Services	Yes	1	1	1	No
Stockport NHS Foundation Trust	Yes	7	5	0	No
Surrey & Sussex Healthcare NHS Trust	Yes	6	4	4	Yes
Tameside Hospital NHS Foundation Trust	Yes	4	2	2	No
Taunton & Somerset NHS Foundation Trust	Yes	6	6	6	Yes
The Christie NHS Foundation Trust	Yes	1	0	0	No
The Queen Elizabeth Hospital King's Lynn NHS Trust	Yes	7	5	5	Yes
The Rotherham NHS Foundation Trust	Yes	4	4	4	Yes
Torbay Care Trust	No	0	0	0	No
Trafford Healthcare NHS Trust	Yes	2	2	1	No
Ulster Independent Clinic	No	0	0	0	Yes
United Bristol Healthcare NHS Trust	Yes	0	0	0	Yes
United Lincolnshire Hospitals NHS Trust	Yes	16	14	10	Yes
Univ. Hospital of South Manchester NHS Foundation Trust	Yes	1	0	0	Yes
University College London Hospitals NHS Foundation Trust	Yes	0	0	0	Yes
University Hospital Birmingham NHS Foundation Trust	Yes	6	6	5	Yes

Participation continued

Organisation	Death data	Clinical Q sent	Clinical Q returned	Casenotes returned	Organis- ational Q returned
University Hospital of North Staffordshire NHS Trust	No	0	0	0	No
University Hospitals Coventry and Warwickshire NHS Trust	Yes	10	10	10	Yes
University Hospitals of Leicester NHS Trust	Yes	14	14	10	Yes
University Hospitals of Morecambe Bay NHS Trust	Yes	9	5	6	Yes
Walsall Hospitals NHS Trust	Yes	8	2	2	No
Waltham Forest Primary Care Trust	No	0	0	0	Yes
Warrington & Halton Hospitals NHS Foundation Trust	Yes	4	2	2	No
West Hertfordshire Hospitals NHS Trust	No	0	0	0	No
West Middlesex University Hospital NHS Trust	Yes	3	0	0	No
West Suffolk Hospitals NHS Trust	Yes	1	1	1	Yes
Western Health & Social Care Trust	No	0	0	0	Yes
Weston Area Health Trust	Yes	3	1	0	No
Whipps Cross University Hospital NHS Trust	Yes	4	3	0	Yes
Whittington Hospital NHS Trust	Yes	4	4	3	Yes
Winchester & Eastleigh Healthcare NHS Trust	Yes	2	1	0	No
Wirral University Teaching Hospital NHS Foundation Trust	Yes	5	5	4	Yes
Worcestershire Acute Hospitals	Yes	18	11	8	Yes
Worthing and Southlands Hospitals NHS Trust	Yes	6	4	1	Yes
Wrightington, Wigan & Leigh NHS Trust	Yes	6	5	4	No
Yeovil District Hospital NHS Foundation Trust	Yes	6	3	2	Yes
York Hospitals NHS Foundation Trust	Yes	4	3	3	Yes

If no death data were reported, this could have been because no deaths occurred during the study period.